Brigitte E. Scammell

ABC OF MAJOR TRAUMA

ABC OF MAJOR TRAUMA

edited by

DAVID SKINNER FRCS

Consultant in accident and emergency medicine, St Bartholomew's Hospital

PETER DRISCOLL FRCS

Consultant in accident and emergency medicine, Whipp's Cross and St Bartholomew's Hospitals

and

RICHARD EARLAM FRCS

Consultant in general surgery, Royal London Hospital

with contributions by

DAVID WATSON, STEPHEN WESTABY, NIGEL BRAYLEY, PETER J F BASKETT,
ROSS BULLOCK, GRAHAM TEASDALE, IAIN HUTCHISON, MICHAEL LAWLOR, ANDREW SWAIN,
JOHN DOVE, HARRY BAKER, ANDREW COPE, WILLIAM STEBBINGS,
TIMOTHY TERRY, ANTHONY DEANE, KEITH M WILLET, HUGH DORRELL, PETER KELLY, N M PERRY,
M D LEWARS, PAMELA NASH, A R LLOYD-THOMAS, I ANDERSON, COLIN ROBERTSON,
OLIVER FENTON, IAN HAYWOOD, ALASTAIR WILSON, STEPHEN MILES, VIRGINIA MURRAY,
C A J McLAUCHLAN, D W YATES

Articles published in
the *British Medical Journal*

Published by the British Medical Journal
Tavistock Square, London WC1H 9JR

First published 1991

British Library Cataloguing in Publication Data

Skinner, David; Driscoll, Peter; and Earlam, Richard
 ABC of major trauma
 1. Man. Trauma. Therapy
 617.1

ISBN 0–7279–0291–1

Printed in Great Britain at the University Press, Cambridge
Typesetting by Bedford Typesetters Ltd, Bedford

Contents

FOREWORD

Ever since the end of the second world war there have been sporadic attempts to draw attention to the enormous problem posed by injury in Western society. Interested individuals have repeatedly pointed out the inadequacy of prehospital, hospital, and rehabilitation services. Calls for remedial action have, at best, elicited only partial responses.

In looking at the statistics, such apparent lack of interest is difficult to understand. Injury is the commonest cause of death among those aged under 35, exceeding the combined deaths caused by cardiovascular disease and cancer. Each week in Britain about 100 people die as a result of accidents on our roads. The 500 000 admissions to hospital each year after injury result in 13 000 hospital beds being occupied each day. The costs to the health service in particular and to society in general are now beginning to be understood. Five per cent of the total health service budget is spent on the management of injury. It is no wonder that injury has been variously described as "the last great plague of the young" and the "neglected epidemic."

Unfortunately, until recently, the medical profession, politicians, the media, and the public have taken little interest in either the prevention or treatment of injury. This is in considerable contrast with some other conditions, such as childhood leukaemia. The media have ensured that wide publicity is given repeatedly to the occasional deaths from leukaemia around Sellafield. In the West Cumbria Health District in the 15 years between 1974 and 1988 eight people under the age of 25 died of leukaemia. It is difficult to know why equal publicity was not given to the 148 people in the same age group who died due to injury over the same period.

Happily, attitudes seem to be changing. In the United Kingdom the new specialty of accident and emergency medicine is now well established. Papers from Germany and North America have emphasised the benefits that can be obtained from high quality prehospital ambulance services and centralising the management of the seriously injured in trauma centres. The publication in 1988 of the report of the Royal College of Surgeons of England on the management of major injuries has led to a thorough reappraisal of the existing services. There is now increased interest and commitment from the major specialties concerned in treating the injured. Advanced trauma life support training has been instituted, and the Department of Health has established the first experimental trauma centre. Thus the publication of this book is timely. It will act as a stimulus to those embarking on a career that includes the assessment and treatment of the injured and will be a valuable reference book for those interested in trauma care.

MILES IRVING

Professor of Surgery,
Hope Hospital,
University of Manchester School of Medicine

December 1990

INTRODUCTION

The management of patients with major injuries in the United Kingdom has been the subject of much discussion and debate over the past five years. The report of the Royal College of Surgeons of England highlighted various areas where medical management was substantially suboptimal; patients who should have survived did not do so because of poor management. The report also emphasised that experienced consultants in various specialties must become more involved in emergency treatment.

The chapter on initial assessment gives a sequential method of management that can be followed by one doctor if he or she is unfortunate enough to be working in isolation. Recent evidence suggests that a "trauma team" approach provides more speedy diagnosis and resuscitation and decreases mortality and morbidity. The same tasks must be completed but they can be allocated to different members of the team in order that the initial assessment is more rapid.

In the instructions on management we and many of the contributors have been influenced by the advanced trauma life support (ATLS) course, as originated by the American College of Surgeons and, more recently, run in the United Kingdom under the auspices of the Royal College of Surgeons of England. We believe that such a system will save lives and therefore have promoted a similar approach.

The various other chapters deal with specific problems related to one part of the body or with particular sorts of injuries, such as burns and blast injuries, or situations where large numbers of casualties are involved. We thank the authors for their efforts in producing a book which will, we hope, be of help to all those treating patients with major trauma. We also thank Fiona Whimster for encouragement and secretarial help.

DAVID SKINNER
PETER DRISCOLL
RICHARD EARLAM

December 1990

INITIAL ASSESSMENT AND MANAGEMENT

Peter Driscoll, David Skinner

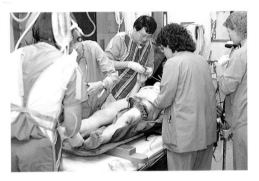

The multiply injured patient has by definition multiple problems, and adequate treatment necessitates a team approach. The team must be organised appropriately and work in a well equipped resuscitation room. The overall management of the patient is the responsibility of the team leader, who should, ideally, not participate in practical procedures but should:
(1) Organise the team
(2) Assimilate the clinical findings and physical measurements
(3) Devise immediate and definitive plans for management.

Objectives of the trauma team

- Identify and correct life threatening injuries
- Resuscitate the patient and stabilise the vital signs
- Determine the extent of other injuries
- Prepare the patient for definitive care, which may mean transporting him or her to another centre

---

Patients with multiple injuries seen in a British accident and emergency department have usually suffered blunt injuries, often caused by road traffic accidents. These patients are difficult to assess because their injuries are not overt. Management of a patient, coordinated by the team leader, will depend on priorities, with attention being paid to identifying and correcting life threatening problems. It is vital that problems should be anticipated and prepared for rather than reacted to.

Before the patient arrives

Responsibilities of members of the trauma team

Team leader—Primary survey; secondary survey; coordinate team effort; overall responsibility for patient while in accident and emergency department

Anaesthetist—Airway control; ventilation; central venous cannulation; fluid balance

Other doctor—All other procedures; chest drain; catheterisation; splintage of fractures; removal of clothes; etc

Nurses (ideally 2)—Measure vital signs; record data; removal of clothes; help doctors; attach monitor

Radiographers—Take specific radiographs of cervical spine, chest, and pelvis in all patients as soon as possible, coordinating with team and other radiographs as clinically necessary

---

Many accident departments are warned of the impending arrival of a patient with multiple injuries by the ambulance service. The team should assemble in the resuscitation room. Each member of the team should wear gloves, a plastic apron, and eye protection.

The trauma team's responsibility is to complete the primary survey and necessary resuscitation and subsequently complete the secondary survey, as well as recording all diagnoses and treatments. The team leader must ensure that this is achieved effectively and rapidly. Ideally, tasks are allocated to different members of the team at an early stage: in a well practised team this can be done even before the patient arrives.

Assessment and resuscitation

Primary survey and resuscitation

Airway and cervical spine control
Breathing
Circulation and haemorrhage control
Dysfunction of the central nervous system
Exposure

Secondary survey

Definitive management

Each patient with multiple injuries should be assessed in the same way. The series of tasks in the box must be performed automatically and simultaneously by the team.

PRIMARY SURVEY

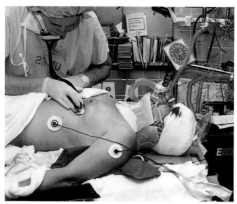

Patient with a rigid collar in place.

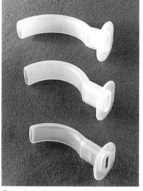

Guedel airways of different sizes.

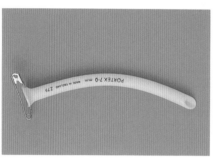

Nasopharyngeal airway. The safety pin prevents inspiration of the airway.

Airway management with protection of the cervical spine

The following activities must not entail moving the neck. Assume that the cervical spine is damaged if there is any suspicion of injury above the clavicles. Keep a rigid cervical collar on the patient unless you are examining the neck, in which case stabilise the cervical spine manually.

Talk to the patient. If he or she replies with a normal voice and gives logical answers to questions the airway is patent and the brain is being perfused adequately. If there is no reply open the patient's mouth and remove any liquid vomit with a rigid sucker. A patient with multiple injuries may have just eaten, and the risk of vomiting is high. Be prepared therefore to suck vomit out immediately. Turning the patient into the recovery position may exacerbate a cervical injury.

The tongue commonly obstructs the airway in unconscious patients, but the airway can be opened by using the chin lift manoeuvre. Remove false teeth and any other solid foreign objects with Magill forceps. Patients who have a gag reflex can maintain their own airway and do not need a Guedel airway, which can precipitate vomiting, cervical movement, and a rise in intracranial pressure. A nasopharyngeal airway is an alternative. If there is no gag reflex the only safe way to ventilate the patient and protect the airway is by using a cuffed endotracheal tube; ventilation with a mask may distend the stomach with air and induce vomiting. During intubation in line stability of the neck must be maintained. Orotracheal rather than nasotracheal intubation is recommended.

Every patient with multiple injuries should receive 100% oxygen.

Having secured the airway, quickly check the neck for swellings, the position of the trachea, and venous distension.

Common causes of inadequate ventilation

Bilateral:
Obstruction of the upper respiratory tract
Leak between the face and mask

Unilateral:
Intubation of the right main bronchus
Pneumothorax
Haemothorax
Lung contusion
Flail segment
Foreign body in main bronchus

Rapid Assessment

Skin colour

Carotid pulse palpable (systolic blood pressure >60 mm Hg)

Femoral pulse palpable (systemic blood pressure >70 mm Hg)

Radial pulse palpable (systolic blood pressure >80 mm Hg)

Breathing

Ensure that both sides of the chest are being ventilated by inspecting for adequate movement and auscultating for breath sounds. Listen particularly in the axilla for ventilation of the periphery of the lung and also over the epigastrium to ensure that the stomach is not being ventilated. Count the respiratory rate.

Circulation and haemorrhage control

Control any major external haemorrhage with direct pressure. Tourniquets are used only when the affected limb is deemed unsalvageable.

The patient's pulse and blood pressure must be recorded, and a cardiac monitor must be attached to the patient.

Two intravenous lines (with needles of gauge 14) should be inserted peripherally. The antecubital fossae are usually the best sites for intravenous infusion, but failing this a cut down may be required. Blood specimens should be taken for determination of group and crossmatch, and for determining full blood count and urea and electrolyte concentrations. A specimen of arterial blood for determination of blood gas tensions should also be taken.

A central line should be inserted primarily for measuring the central venous pressure. If a chest drain is already in place the central line should be inserted on the same side. Changes in the central venous pressure are more important than individual measurements.

A colloid solution is usually given in the first instance to maintain the fluid balance, and if there are any signs of hypovolaemia 1 litre should be given rapidly while the vital signs are being monitored. The need for further fluids and their rate of flow are determined by the vital signs. Blood is required after a major injury or when there has been a limited response to 2 litres of colloid. Blood should be warmed before use. The pneumatic anti-shock garment has been shown to be useful in shocked patients, particularly those suspected of having fractures of the pelvis and legs.

> Changes in the central venous pressure are more important than individual measurements

> If a life threatening problem is identified during this rapid primary survey it must be corrected immediately rather than waiting until the end of the survey. For example, a tension pneumothorax must be treated on discovery

Dysfunction of the central nervous system

A rapid assessment of the brain and spinal cord is made by assessing the pupils and by asking patients to put their tongue out, wiggle their toes, and squeeze your fingers. The more detailed Glasgow coma scale assessment is then carried out.

Exposure

By this stage all clothing should have been removed. Movement should be kept to an absolute minimum, which means that clothing has to be cut away with a large sharp pair of scissors. Do not, however, allow the patient to get cold: the resuscitation room should be warm and the patient covered when not being examined.

SECONDARY SURVEY

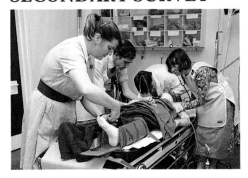

The following scheme describes how to perform a detailed head to toe examination of the patient. In addition, it should be standard practice to perform lateral cervical spine, chest, and pelvic radiography in patients with blunt trauma. Protective lead aprons should be worn by staff who continue to manage the patient. One doctor, who may be the team leader, should be responsible for the secondary survey; the examination should be orderly and complete.

Head and neck

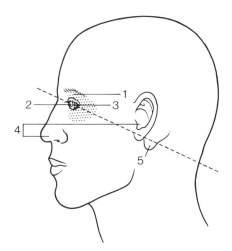

1—Racoon eyes (bilateral periorbital haematoma)
2—Subhyaloid haemorrhage
3—Scleral haemorrhage without a posterior margin
4—Haemotympanium
 —Cerebrospinal fluid rhinorrhoea and otorrhoea
5—Battle's sign (bruising over the mastoid process)

Scalp

Palpate from posterior to anterior. Check for lacerations, swellings, and depressions. Palpate for fractures at the base of lacerations. Profuse bleeding of the scalp must be stopped.

Neurological state

The patient's level of consciousness must be monitored regularly and recorded according to the Glasgow coma scale. As the score for motor response varies among hospitals (some using a maximum score of 14 and others 15) describe the findings as well as giving the score. **Deterioration may not be due to the primary injury to the brain but may reflect hypoxia or hypoperfusion.**

Base of skull

Externally the base of the skull runs from the mastoid process to the orbit. Consequently, fractures of the basal skull may produce signs along this line.

When there is cerebrospinal fluid rhinorrhoea or otorrhoea the fluid is invariably mixed with blood, and this will delay the clotting of the blood and produce a double ring pattern if dropped on to a sheet. Examination with an auroscope may precipitate meningitis in patients with such problems.

Eyes

Examine the eyes early, before orbital swelling makes this impossible. Look for haemorrhages inside or outside, foreign bodies under the lids, and any signs of penetrating injuries. Visual acuity can be tested rapidly by asking the patient to read a label. If the patient is unconscious test the pupillary response and the corneal reflex.

Face

The face should be palpated symmetrically for deformities and tenderness. Check for loose or lost teeth. Grasp the upper incisors and determine whether there is any instability of the maxilla, which would suggest a middle third fracture. These fractures may be associated with fractures of the basal skull. Only those fractures compromising the airway need to be treated immediately. This may entail pulling the fractured facial skeleton segment forwards to clear the airway.

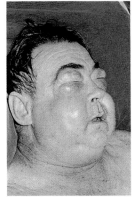

Extreme facial oedema.

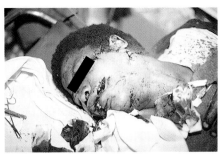

Facial injury likely to obstruct the airway.

Initial assessment and management

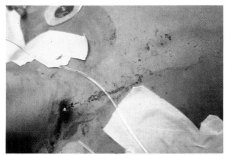
Gunshot wound in the neck.

Neck

With the head held firmly by an assistant undo the cervical collar and examine the neck. Look for any deformity, bruising, or lacerations. Palpate each of the cervical spinous processes to detect tenderness and "step off" deformities. Palpate the posterior cervical neck muscles for spasm and tenderness. Conscious patients will also assist by telling you if there is any pain in the neck and, if so, its location. Inspect lacerations of the neck, and if the wound penetrates the platysma it needs to be explored under general anaesthesia in the operating theatre. A lateral cervical spine radiograph showing all seven cervical vertebrae is essential in patients with multiple injuries. The patient's arms should be pulled towards the feet while the radiograph is being taken. Remember that this radiograph can miss fractures of C1 and C2 and the low cervical vertebrae. An anteroposterior radiograph of the cervical spine and odontoid peg is required for full evaluation of the cervical spine, but this can be delayed until the secondary survey has been completed.

Thorax

Immediately life threatening thoracic injuries

Obstruction of the airway
Open chest wound
Tension pneumothorax
Massive haemopneumothorax
Cardiac tamponade

The priority at this stage is to identify conditions that are immediately or potentially life threatening. Immediately life threatening injuries must be treated when found.

Inspect the chest for bruising, wounds, signs of respiratory obstruction, and asymmetry of movement. Forces of acceleration and deceleration can produce extensive thoracic injuries, but they often leave marks on the chest wall. Certain patterns may be associated with particular types of injury. The bruise resulting from pressure exerted by a diagonal seat belt may overlay a fractured clavicle, a tear in the thoracic aorta, pulmonary contusion, and a lacerated pancreas. The mark caused by impact with the central steering wheel suggests a sternal fracture with cardiac contusion.

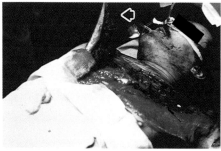
Open sucking chest wound.

Lung and chest wall

A flail segment is diagnosed when paradoxical movement of a segment of the chest wall is observed. Small flail segments are difficult to diagnose and require careful inspection of the chest wall. Immediate treatment of this condition may be necessary, depending on the degree of underlying contusion of the lung. If analysis of the blood gases shows a low PO_2 or if the patient is becoming exhausted intubation and intermittent positive pressure ventilation are necessary.

An open chest wound must be covered with an occlusive dressing. A chest drain must then be inserted into the affected side of the chest to prevent the development of a tension pneumothorax.

Palpate the chest by feeling the ribs in the apices of both axillae. Feel for crepitus and tenderness in conscious patients. Continue in a caudal manner. Palpate the anterior aspect of the chest by pressing on both clavicles, each rib, and the sternum. Note the presence of surgical emphysema. Squeeze the chest in a lateral and anteroposterior plane to detect the presence of multiple rib fractures.

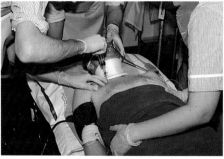
Needle aspiration of a potential pneumothorax.

Auscultation detects differences in air entry between the two sides of the chest. Even in the presence of a pneumothorax air entry can sometimes be heard over the anterior aspect of the chest, especially if the patient is being ventilated. Always listen peripherally for a difference in air entry; a significant difference suggests a pneumothorax, which, if under tension, needs immediate drainage. To do this insert a large bore intravenous cannula in the second intercostal space in the mid-clavicular line on the affected side. A sudden release of air confirms the diagnosis. If there is no release of air perform radiography of the chest immediately to confirm the diagnosis before inserting the chest drain. A pneumothorax or haemothorax should be treated by inserting a chest drain with a gauge of >28 in the fifth intercostal space just anterior to the mid-axillary line. This enables air and fluid to be drained.

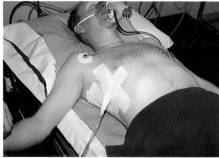
Chest drain in situ.

Other potentially life threatening conditions (for example, dissecting aortic aneurysm, ruptured oesophagus, and ruptured diaphragm) must be identified at this stage. Their detailed management is described in the chapter on thoracic trauma.

Heart

The mechanism of injury will often indicate the possibility of damage to the cardiac or thoracic aorta. Invariably the signs will be subtle. Patients with extreme physical signs usually die at the scene of the accident. Cardiac contusion should be suspected if the chest has been subjected to a decelerating force, such as a fall from a height or road traffic accident. This may produce sternal bruising and tenderness. Cardiac arrhythmias or an infarction pattern seen on the cardiac monitor may reflect cardiac contusion. Rapid deceleration forces may also produce a tear in the thoracic aorta.

Penetrating thoracic injuries may damage the heart and produce pericardial tamponade. The classic features of this condition may not be present in a patient with multiple injuries. In view of the diagnostic difficulty doctors should have a low threshold for performing a percutaneous pericardial aspiration. This will also relieve the problem temporarily.

Circulation

The degree of hypovolaemic shock is estimated by noting the patient's skin colour, pulse, pulse volume, and blood pressure. Up to a 30% loss of blood volume will produce a tachycardia and decreased pulse pressure, but the blood pressure may remain within normal limits. A consistent fall in the systolic blood pressure will occur only when more than 30% of the blood volume has been lost. A urine output of less than 50 ml/h in an adult indicates poor renal perfusion, suggesting poor perfusion of the tissues in general.

The adequacy of fluid resuscitation is measured by the same variables. One of three responses may be seen:

(1) The vital signs return to normal after infusion of less than 1 litre of colloid solution. In such cases patients have lost less than 20% of their blood volume and are not actively bleeding.

(2) The vital signs initially improve with the infusion but then deteriorate. In such cases patients are actively bleeding and have usually lost more than 20% of their blood volume. They need to be transfused with typed blood, and the source of bleeding must be controlled; this may require an operation.

(3) The vital signs do not improve at all. This suggests that either the shock has not been caused by hypovolaemia or the patient is actively bleeding faster than fluid is being infused. History, mechanism of injury, and physical findings (including the central venous pressure) will help to distinguish between these two possibilities. Blood can be crossmatched urgently in 15 minutes or less in most laboratories. Transfusion of group O negative blood is justified only when crossmatching is not available.

Patients with hypovolaemia whose vital signs do not improve at all have usually lost over 40% of their blood volume. The source of bleeding is invariably in the thorax, abdomen, or pelvis and requires an operation to correct it.

Signs of pericardial tamponade

Beck's triad

1 Jugular venous pressure raised
2 Muffled heart sounds
3 Blood pressure reduced

Pulsus paradoxicus

Pulse rate raised

Hypovolaemic shock

Skin colour
Pulse
Pulse volume
Blood pressure

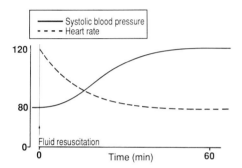

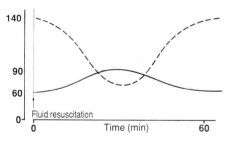

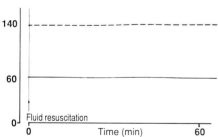

Abdomen

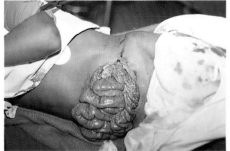

Eviseration of the bowel after an abdominal wound.

Inspect the abdomen for bruising, movement, and wounds. Cover any exposed bowel with a sterile pack soaked in warm saline. Explore any laceration; if it extends into muscle the wound must be formally explored at laparotomy.

Initial assessment and management

Palpate for tenderness and note any signs of urethral injury in men. Squeezing the pelvis in two planes will detect only severe abnormalities. Every patient with multiple injuries must undergo pelvic radiography and rectal examination. The importance of bowel sounds is controversial; decisions on abdominal management should never rely solely on the presence or absence of bowel sounds.

Intra-abdominal bleeding should be suspected if there are fractures of ribs 5-11, which lie over the liver and spleen, or if there are marks caused by seat belts or tyres over the abdomen.

A catheter must be inserted so that the patient's rate of urine output can be measured. A per-urethral approach is used if there is no evidence of urethral injury. If urethral damage is suspected a suprapubic catheter should be inserted, and subsequently a retrograde urethrogram will be required. The urine must be tested for blood. If the result is positive a one shot intravenous pyelogram can be taken in the resuscitation room. This will show whether both kidneys are present, functioning, and with or without major disruption. This rapid investigation is usually performed on a patient going for an urgent operation, when the presence of any major renal disease needs to be excluded. If there is no urgency a definitive intravenous pyelogram and cystogram can be performed at the end of the examination. Urine should be saved for possible future microscopical examination and analysis of drug concentrations.

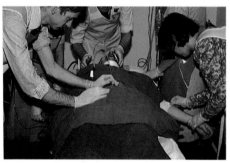

Patient undergoing peritoneal lavage.

Occasionally there is pronounced gastric distension. A nasogastric tube decompresses the stomach and facilitates the examination of the abdomen.

Abdominal palpation may be unreliable, particularly in a patient with a head injury or one who is drunk. A diagnostic peritoneal lavage will rule out intraperitoneal injury in such a patient. The general surgeon who will be looking after the patient must be present while this procedure is undertaken.

Extremities

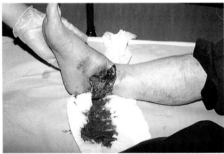

Compound fracture and dislocation of the right ankle.

Inspect the arms and legs for bruising, wounds, and deformities. In all patients check distal pulses and sensation. The viability of the skin overlying a fracture or dislocation must be assessed. Correct limb deformities and recheck peripheral pulses and sensation. Do all of this before performing radiography on the area as delays can result in loss of tissue. Palpate and rotate all long bones, noting any crepitus and instability. Test for active movement if the patient is conscious. Swabs should be taken for microbiological analysis from sites of compound fracture and wounds then covered with a sterile dressing. Splint all fractures: this will inhibit movement, reducing further damage to soft tissues and possible production of fat emboli as well as reducing pain. A polaroid picture taken before covering a compound fracture will prevent repeated inspection and decrease the risk of infection.

Spinal column

Spinal injuries can be partial or complete. Test for sensory and motor defects and note any degree of priapism; the penis does not have to be fully erect for this condition to be diagnosed. The results of these tests indicate the level and extent of damage. If the cord has been transected above the level of the sympathetic outflow hypotension without tachycardia results. The degree of vasodilatation producing spinal shock depends on how much sympathetic tone remains. Transection of the cervical spinal cord removes all vasoconstrictor tone and consequently produces profound hypotension.

If there is evidence of a spinal cord injury the patient should not be moved. Do not turn the patient to examine the back as this can increase the degree of neurological damage if the vertebral column is unstable. Radiographs of the affected sites are required initially so that management can be planned. The exceptions to the rule of not turning patients are those with penetrating injuries in whom the exit wound is not visible.

> **If you suspect a spinal injury do not move the patient**

Back

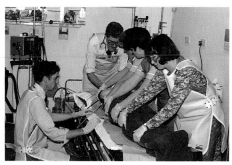

Log rolling a patient to enable examination of the back.

If there is no damage to the spinal cord the patient can be log rolled and the whole of the back examined. The patient should be turned away from the team leader so that the debris under the patient can be cleared away and the back inspected. Look for bruising and open wounds and auscultate the back of the chest. Inspect between the buttocks for the exit or entry site of a penetrating injury. "Walk" down the vertebral column with your fingers, feeling for boggyness, malalignment, and step off deformities. Remember that patients can have vertebral column injuries without these signs. Sites of tenderness in conscious patients must be recorded. Finally, palpate the longitudinal spinal muscles for spasm and tenderness. The patient is then log rolled back into the supine position.

Medical history

> **Assessment of patient**
>
> A Allergies
> M Medicines
> P Past medical history
> L Last meal
> E Events leading to the injury

This should now be assessed. Information may be available from the patient, relatives, and the ambulance crew. A useful mnemonic is given in the box.

Further x ray films may now be taken. Clearly, this should not precede or interfere with management of life threatening conditions—a ruptured spleen should be operated on before radiological confirmation of a fractured metacarpal.

Reassessment

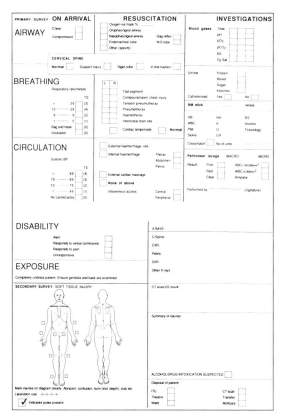

Pages two and three of the trauma sheet.

The team leader must constantly evaluate the response to resuscitation:

(1) Is the patient improving, deteriorating, or unchanged since resuscitation started? If the patient is not improving then recheck the results of the Airway, Breathing, and Circulation investigations of the primary survey. The patient's condition can change rapidly: repeated examination and constant monitoring are essential.

(2) What is the extent of the injuries and what are the priorities for treatment?

(3) Has an injury been missed? If you have not found an injury in a body cavity between two injured sites you have probably missed it. Re-examine the patient.

(4) What is the patient's tetanus state, and are antibiotics required?

(5) Patients with multiple injuries require pain relief. A mixture of 50% nitrous oxide and 50% oxygen (Entonox) should be given until the baseline observations are recorded. Morphine can then be given intravenously, the dose being determined by titration against the patient's response.

The team leader is responsible for all documentation, which must be accurate and complete, and should write up the case notes. If a criminal cause of injury is suspected all clothes, loose debris, bullets, etc, should be bagged, labelled, and signed.

Responsibility for continuing care should be formally handed over, usually to the senior duty general surgeon, when the patient leaves the accident and emergency department.

The photograph of the Guedel airway was taken by Ashworth Assaye, *BMJ* department of medical illustration. The photographs depicting periorbital oedema, facial injury, and a penetrating neck injury were reproduced from the advanced trauma life support™ (ATLS™) slide set by kind permission of the American College of Surgeons' committee on trauma. The line drawing of the head was prepared by the department of education and medical illustration services, St Bartholomew's Hospital, who also supplied the photograph of a trauma team at work.

MANAGEMENT OF THE UPPER AIRWAY

David Watson

First vital minutes

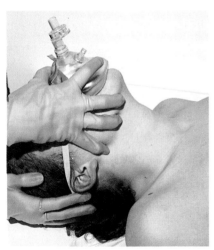

Mouth-to-face mask.

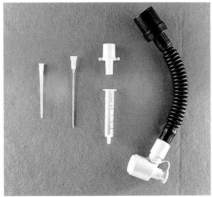

Apparatus for needle cricothyroidotomy. Modified large bore intravenous cannula and anaesthetic connections.

All severely injured patients have hypoxaemia in varying degrees. As soon as medical help arrives the first priority must be to ensure that the patient's airway is free and ventilation is unimpaired. Immediate administration of supplementary oxygen to the unobstructed airway is of paramount importance. Remember that in the first vital minutes the cervical spine of any patient with trauma should be considered broken until proved otherwise. The neck must be kept stabilised without traction (for example by using a spine board, sand bags, or a hard collar) at all times until the possibility of neck injury is excluded.

In an unconscious patient any obstruction to the airway must be removed under direct vision. The laryngeal and pharyngeal reflexes should then be assessed and respiratory performance examined. If protective reflexes are adequate—for example, the patient is coughing—retracting the tongue foward by employing the chin lift or jaw thrust manoeuvre or inserting an anaesthetic type airway or nasopharyngeal tube may suffice. If the reflexes are depressed or absent—that is, there is no gag reflex when oropharyngeal suction is attempted in an unconscious patient—the airway must be secured at the earliest opportunity by intubation with an appropriately sized endotracheal tube with a low pressure cuff.

Patients with hypoxia or apnoea must be ventilated and oxygenated before intubation is attempted. Ventilation can be achieved with a mouth-to-face mask or bag-valve-face mask. Studies suggest that ventilation techniques with a bag-valve-face-mask are less effective when performed by one person rather than two people, when one of the pair can use both hands to assure a good seal. When only one person is present to provide ventilation the method employing the mouth-to-face mask is preferred. During such manoeuvres the neck must be kept immobilised.

If intubation is performed a large bore gastric tube should also be passed. Nasal passage of a gastric tube is contraindicated in patients with suspected basal skull fractures or injury to the cribriform plate.

Tracheostomy is rarely necessary as an emergency procedure. Severe distorting injury to the structures above or at the level of the larynx can render endotracheal intubation impossible, but cricothyroidotomy—for example, with a large bore intravenous cannula—is preferred to emergency tracheostomy in such circumstances.

In patients with fractured ribs with or without a pneumothorax chest drainage on the side of the fractures is mandatory before artificial ventilation is undertaken. A tension pneumothorax should always be suspected when a patient with a recent crush injury has obvious respiratory distress or cyanosis. In patients with a chest injury complicated by pneumothorax an apical chest drain should be inserted through the space between the fifth and sixth ribs, just anterior to the midaxillary line. If there is blood in the pleural cavity an additional basal drain may be required.

An open pneumothorax should be managed initially by occluding the open wound with a petroleum jelly gauze or other non-porous dressing. A chest tube is also inserted to relieve any accumulated air and prevent the development of a tension pneumothorax.

Indications for oxygenation and ventilation

> • Ventilatory assistance is required when there is excessive respiratory work or obvious ventilatory insufficiency
> • Failure of adequate oxygenation ($P_aO_2 < 9$ kPa) when the patient is breathing a high inspired oxygen concentration (6 l/min O_2 by facemask) demands endotracheal intubation and assisted positive pressure ventilation

Once the airway is secured the adequacy of the exchange of respiratory gases must be evaluated. The respiratory rate can be counted and respiratory effort assessed. Measurements of blood gas tensions should be undertaken as soon as is practicable.

Artificial ventilation in patients without respiratory failure must also be considered when there is coincidental head injury. Hypercapnia and hypoxaemia from asphyxia or inadequate ventilation with fluctuations in arterial blood pressure cause considerable deterioration in cerebral function. This is probably secondary to alterations in cerebral blood flow that adversely affect intracranial pressure.

Hospital management

> ### Intubation of patients with head injuries
> • Assume the patient has a cervical fracture
> • An anaesthetist performs laryngoscopy while an assistant holds the patient's head
> • Pressure on the cricoid must be provided by an assistant to prevent aspiration of gastric contents

An anaesthetist experienced in caring for victims of trauma should be available to examine the patient immediately on arrival at hospital. Evaluation of the patient's airway must proceed simultaneously with treatment. If the airway is satisfactory treatment may consist simply of increased oxygen delivery. If the airway is comprised or the patient needs ventilatory support a secure intratracheal airway, if not already in place, is required. Patients with hypoxia or apnoea must be ventilated and oxygenated before intubation is attempted.

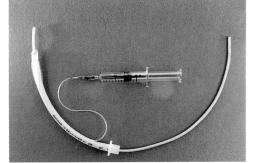

Gum elastic bougie and endotracheal tube.

The route of choice for securing the airway depends on several factors. Blunt trauma of the head and face is associated with an incidence of fractures of the cervical spine of 5 to 10%.[1] Patients with trauma should be assumed to have a cervical fracture until proved otherwise; manipulation of the neck is strictly contraindicated. Doctors in the United Kingdom generally accept that laryngoscopy and orotracheal intubation after induction of anaesthesia and muscle paralysis can be performed by a competent operator with minimal changes in the position of the cervical vertebrae while an assistant holds the patient's head. Although optimum exposure of the larynx is not achievable under such conditions, experienced anaesthetists can intubate patients without clearly visualising the vocal cords. This may require aids such as the gum elastic bougie. Pressure on the cricoid must be provided by a skilled assistant to protect the patient from aspirating gastric contents.[2] The stomach may already have been emptied as much as possible by the passage of a nasogastric tube with the neck immobilised.

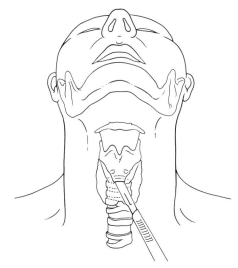

Cricothyroidotomy with scalpel.

Tracheostomy may be necessary for patients who cannot be intubated either nasally or orally. Often these patients have massive facial trauma. Although surgical cricothyroidotomy can be performed through a small midline incision in the cricothyroid membrane, life saving oxygenation can also be provided by needle cricothyroidotomy with a cannula connected to an anaesthetic circuit for assisted ventilation. Spontaneous respiration after needle cricothyroidotomy, however, can be extremely difficult, requiring large pressure changes in the airway and considerable ventilatory effort. Assisted ventilation with sedation and muscle paralysis is therefore necessary.

Anaesthetic considerations

Anaesthetists caring for patients who are critically ill reduce the doses of all anaesthetics because hypovolaemia and hypotension alter the distribution and pharmacokinetics of drugs, thereby exaggerating their clinical effects. Opiates and barbiturates are therefore given in smaller doses to avoid cardiovascular depression. Ketamine and halogenated hydrocarbons such as halothane raise intracranial pressure and are contraindicated in trauma of the head. Ketamine (1 to 2 mg/kg) and partial opiate agonists such as nalbuphine, however, are useful in trauma that is complicated by haemorrhagic shock. Muscle relaxants given to facilitate intubation include suxamethonium (1·0 mg/kg), pancuronium (0·1 to 0·2 mg/kg), vecuronium (0·1 to 0·2 mg/kg) or atracurium (0·4 mg/kg). Often patients have taken drugs such as opiates, cocaine, and marijuana before suffering trauma. These may interact with anaesthetics. Ethanol enhances the effect of anaesthetics and sedatives and reduces the minimum alveolar concentration of volatile general anaesthetics required.[3]

Before embarking on intubation an anaesthetist will check the equipment, including the suction and oxygen delivery apparatus. Anaesthetics should be ready in labelled syringes, and duplicate ampoules should be easily accessible. Vasoactive drugs such as atropine should also be ready in syringes in case untoward bradycardia complicates extended laryngoscopy. A skilled assistant must be at hand to apply pressure on the cricoid. The neck must be kept stabilised. Secure venous access is mandatory.

Anaesthesia is induced only after administration of oxygen with the best possible monitoring available. Pressure on the cricoid is maintained by the assistant. Neuromuscular blockade is produced by suxamethonium, and intubation proceeds with the onset of paralysis and relaxation of the jaw.

Patients with responsive airway reflexes require induction of anaesthesia and muscle paralysis for the airway to be secured by either an oral or a nasotracheal route. Deeply unconscious patients with trauma of the head and brain injury should not be intubated without prior administration of a cerebral sedative and muscle relaxant, hence avoiding dangerous increases in cerebral blood volume and intracranial pressure during laryngoscopy. Nasotracheal intubation should not be undertaken if fractures of the base of the skull or of the cribriform plate are suspected.

Intubation technique

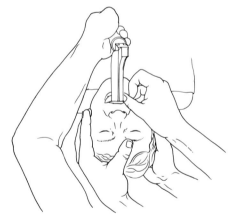

Inserting the laryngoscope.

The anaesthetist takes the laryngoscope in his or her left hand and inserts it into the right hand side of the patient's mouth, thereby moving the tongue to the left. While carefully observing the back of the tongue he or she advances the curved blade of the laryngoscope until the epiglottis comes into view.

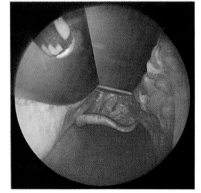

Lifting the root of the tongue.

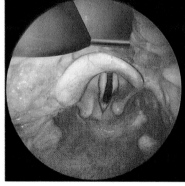

Direct visualisation of the glottis.

The tip of the blade is moved anterior to the epiglottis and the whole lower jaw lifted upwards, taking care not to move the neck. This should expose the arytenoid cartilages and vocal cords. The tracheal rings should be visible beyond. Under direct vision the anaesthetist advances a 60 cm gum elastic bougie or the endotracheal tube, aiming for the left vocal cord. If a gum elastic bougie is used a cut cuffed endotracheal tube of the appropriate size is subsequently "rail roaded" into the trachea. A size 8 tube is usually suitable for women and a size nine for men. The cuff of the endotracheal tube is then inflated with air from a syringe until an airtight seal is secured. The chest should be auscultated in both axillae to exclude intubation of the right main bronchus or oesophagus. Pressure on the cricoid can only now be released and the tube secured with tapes.

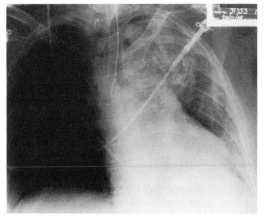

Chest radiograph showing inadvertent intubation of the right main bronchus.

The photographs of ventilation, the apparatus for needle cricothyroidotomy, and the gum elastic bougie were taken by Ashworth Assaye, medical illustration department, *BMJ*. The illustrations of the technique of intubation were reproduced from *A Systematic Guide to Intubation* (by P Lotz, F W Annefeld, and W K Hirlinger) by kind permission of the publisher, Atelier Flad, Eckental, West Germany, and the line drawings were prepared by the education and medical illustration services department, St Bartholomew's Hospital.

After intubation ventilation should proceed with a tidal volume of about 10 ml/kg at a rate of about 10 breaths each minute. Analysis of arterial blood gases should be undertaken at the first opportunity to reassess oxygenation and the adequacy of ventilation. Radiography of the chest should also be performed routinely after endotracheal intubation to catalogue the position of the endotracheal tube in the bronchial tree.

In conclusion, providing oxygen and ventilatory support as early as possible are prerequisites for successful resuscitation in victims of major trauma. Otherwise, as Haldane observed, hypoxia not only stops the machine but wrecks the machinery.

1 McCabe JB, Angelos MG. Injury to the head and face in patients with cervical spine injury. *Am J Emerg Med* 1984;2:333.
2 Sellick BA. Cricoid pressure to control regurgitation of stomach contents during induction of anaesthesia. *Lancet* 1961;ii:404.
3 Bruce DL. Alcoholism and anesthesia. *Anesth Analg* 1983;62:84.

THORACIC TRAUMA

Stephen Westaby, Nigel Brayley

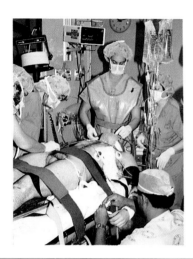

Many patients with catastrophic intrathoracic visceral injury such as laceration of the heart, aorta, or major airways die at the site of incident. Those who reach hospital alive are a self selected group who should survive with early skilled intervention. Yet evidence suggests that most patients who die in hospital of thoracic trauma do so unnecessarily through lack of appropriate treatment. In practice, less than 15 per cent of patients with chest injuries require surgical intervention, pathology in the remainder being confined to the thoracic cage and underlying lung parenchyma. Multiple rib fractures with pulmonary contusion, haemothorax, or pneumothorax can be dealt with simply and effectively by insertion of a chest drain, pain relief, fluid restriction, and physiotherapy. When ignored, underestimated, or inadequately treated, however, such injuries may cause death during surgery for seemingly more important intracranial or abdominal haemorrhage. The basis for successful management of thoracic trauma is effective cardiopulmonary resuscitation followed by early detection and correction of life threatening injuries.

Mechanisms and patterns of blunt thoracic trauma

Chest wall injuries	Possible thoracic visceral injuries	Common associated injuries
High velocity impact (deceleration)		
Chest wall often intact or fractured sternum or bilateral rib fractures with anterior flail (caused by steering wheel)	Ruptured aorta Cardiac contusion Major airways injury Ruptured diaphragm	Head and faciomaxillary injuries Fractured cervical spine Lacerated liver or spleen Long bone fractures
Low velocity impact (direct blow)		
Lateral—unilateral fractured ribs	Pulmonary contusion	Lacerated liver or spleen if ribs 6-12 are fractured
Anterior—fractured sternum	Cardiac contusion	
Crush		
Anteroposterior—bilateral rib fractures with or without anterior flail	Ruptured bronchus Cardiac contusion	Fractured thoracic spine Lacerated liver or spleen
Lateral—ipsilateral fractures with or without flail Possible contralateral fractures	Pulmonary contusion	Lacerated liver or spleen

Reception and general assessment of the multiply injured patient have been dealt with in previous articles in this series. It is imperative to determine within the first few minutes whether an immediately life threatening thoracic problem exists. The primary survey must take into account the mechanism of injury: there are distinct patterns of injury according to whether the patient has suffered high velocity, low velocity, crush, or penetrating trauma. Remember that the most serious intrathoracic injuries can occur without damage to the chest wall. Diagnosis may be difficult and should depend on prediction and exclusion rather than direct manifestation of injury.

Immediately life threatening pathophysiological processes

- *Hypoxia and acidosis* secondary to major airway obstruction, haemopneumothorax, pulmonary contusion, or a major circulatory disorder. Is the patient blue, tachypnoeic, cerebrally obtunded, sweaty, or cold?
- *Low cardiac output* secondary to haemorrhage in the chest or abdomen, cardiac tamponade, or profound metabolic deterioration. Does the patient's colour, vital signs, and peripheral perfusion suggest this? Is there active bleeding?
- *Cardiac or vascular injury* that may prove fatal during resuscitation

When the thoracic cage and underlying lungs are injured hypoxia and acidosis caused by untreated haemopneumothorax compound the effects of a direct head injury and should be resolved quickly. Generally, major injuries such as aortic transection, major airways disruption, diaphragmatic rupture, and serious cardiac disruption are apparent in the plain chest radiograph. Such radiography should be undertaken as part of the primary survey and certainly before radiography of the abdomen or limbs. Remember that cardiac or major vascular lacerations with haemorrhage arrested by tamponade may rapidly become fatal during transfusion and raising of intracardiac or arterial pressures. If such injuries are not identified before full resuscitation the patient may bleed to death rapidly as normal blood pressure is restored.

Analysis of blood gas tensions and chest radiography should be undertaken within the first 10 minutes after hospital admission in any patient in whom an important chest injury is suspected.

Decide whether the clinical findings are those expected from the mechanism of injury. Determine whether the chest injury is more life threatening than associated head or abdominal injuries. From the physical examination determine whether the patient is in immediate danger or whether it is safe to proceed with computed tomography or further radiological assessment of other systems.

In multiply injured patients with head injury, haemothorax, and intra-abdominal bleeding it is imperative to resuscitate the brain and myocardium. Not infrequently the patient is moribund from cardiac tamponade, upper airways obstruction, tension haemopneumothorax, or profound haemorrhage. Securing the airway by endotracheal intubation or bronchoscopy, evacuation of haemopneumothorax by insertion of a chest drain, or, in the event of tamponade or torrential haemorrhage, immediate thoracotomy must be undertaken on the basis of physical findings.

In the absence of perceptible blood pressure left anterolateral thoracotomy through the fifth interspace can be undertaken to clamp the descending aorta and perform internal cardiac massage. This facilitates restoration of perfusion pressure to the brain and coronary arteries while arresting intra-abdominal haemorrhage. If present, cardiac tamponade can be relieved. With restoration of cardiac output to the upper part of body requirement for craniotomy must be determined rapidly, before performing abdominal surgery. Remember that in the presence of potentially lethal brain, cardiac, or aortic injury other injuries are of secondary importance.

Resuscitation

Appropriate intervention in patients requiring resuscitation must be based on the immediately life threatening problem but follows the ABC of resuscitation principle, beginning with intubation and positive pressure ventilation if required. Securing a reliable airway may be particularly hazardous in patients who have sustained blunt or penetrating trauma to the root of the neck or upper chest. If laryngeal or tracheal disruption is suspected in a patient who is breathing spontaneously blind intubation may prove fatal and must give way to expert bronchoscopic negotiation of the airway. This is preferable to tracheostomy in advance of accurate definition of the nature of injury. With complete tracheal transection immediate collar incision with location of the distal trachea may be necessary.

Early correction of hypoxia and acidosis are of paramount importance, particularly in the presence of head injury or when urgent surgery for abdominal injuries must be undertaken. This can be done only on the basis of blood gas tensions and acid-base analyses. When hypoxia and acidosis are confirmed one or more of the following steps are necessary.

- Improve the mechanics of breathing by clearing major airways obstruction or draining a haemopneumothorax. Alleviate pain from fractured ribs or undertake mechanical ventilation if the severity of chest wall disruption and pulmonary disruption so demands
- Improve oxygen transport by increasing the inspired oxygen content. Restrict the amount of clear fluid infused and restore the circulating oxygen carrying capacity by blood transfusion after profuse haemorrhage
- Improve the circulation and oxygen delivery by arresting haemorrhage, restoring circulating blood volume, relieving cardiac tamponade, and giving calcium or inotropes if necessary. Before restoring the systolic blood pressure to >100 mg Hg rule out potentially catastrophic cardiac or aortic laceration and potentially fatal secondary haemorrhage.

Thoracic trauma

Accurate assessment and correction of acid-base balance, derangement of blood gas tensions, and the circulatory state require early insertion of central venous and radial arterial lines. Only then can improvement or deterioration in condition during the first hour of resuscitation be monitored sensibly and pharmacological intervention be assessed.

Penetrating wounds

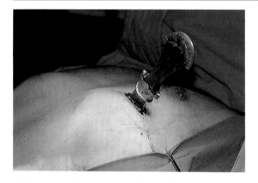

Knife wound in the chest. The knife moved with the cardiac cycle.

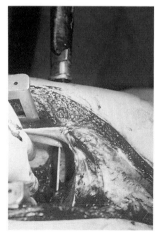

The knife transfixed the pericardium and lacerated but did not penetrate the inferior surface of the heart. The patient left hospital after four days.

Most penetrating wounds damage only the chest wall and underlying lung. In many wounds haemorrhage has already stopped by the time the patient reaches hospital. Insertion of an intercostal drain with suction is all that is required. The necessity for surgical intervention is based on the rate of bleeding or leakage of air from the intercostal drain. Cardiac tamponade, a transmediastinal missile track, and injury to the major airways or oesophagus are definite indications for thoracotomy. Suspected oesophageal or major airways involvement should be investigated by endoscopy beforehand to determine the precise site of injury. False aneurysms from major vessel laceration are delineated by digital subtraction angiography.

When patients are admitted with knives or transfixing implements still in place no attempt should be made to remove these until the surgeon is satisfied that no major vascular structure is damaged or until the patient is in position for thoracotomy; even then it is wise to leave the implement in situ until thoracotomy has exposed the damaged structures.

Patients with penetrating wounds that damage the aorta or main pulmonary arteries usually die before reaching hospital, as do those with appreciable disruption of the atria or ventricles. In contrast, patients with simple stab wounds that affect the heart but not a major coronary artery usually reach hospital alive with cardiac tamponade and their injuries are easily remediable by immediate or early sternotomy and repair. Until a cardiac or vascular injury is ruled out do not raise the systemic pressure uncontrollably as this may precipitate bleeding and death. A central venous and a large bore peripheral cannula should be inserted in preparation for rapid transfusion during the operation.

Cardiopulmonary bypass is rarely required in patients with penetrating thoracic trauma. Consequently, if a hospital does not have cardiothoracic surgeons either the general surgeon must be prepared to intervene or, if time allows, a thoracic surgeon should be transferred from the nearest regional centre. Interhospital transfer of patients with serious penetrating thoracic injuries is contraindicated.

Pericardiocentesis

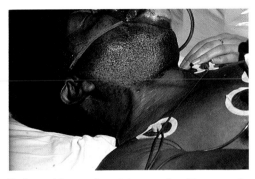

Patient with a cardiac stab wound and tamponade. The neck veins are greatly distended despite blood loss.

Pericardiocentesis may be life saving in extreme circumstances but has caused death through cardiac laceration. It is therefore important that the procedure is performed with skill and caution by an adequately trained surgeon. In cardiac tamponade there is a fine balance between internal and external cardiac pressures that prevents exsanguination. The blood within the pericardium is usually clotted and cannot be aspirated. If the patient is moribund immediate thoracotomy is more important than attempted pericardial aspiration. Such aspiration may sometimes be undertaken on diagnostic grounds when two dimensional echocardiography is not immediately available. After the patient has been attached to an electrocardiographic monitor a transdiaphragmatic approach is undertaken by inserting a wide bore needle of at least 15 cm length from a site between the xiphisternum and left costal margin, aiming the tip of the needle cautiously towards the base of the pericardium along the line of the left sternal margin. The syringe is carefully aspirated during the course of inserting the needle until either altered blood rapidly fills it or the myocardium can be felt on the tip of the needle. Serious laceration of the right or left ventricles is unusual, though damage to the posterior descending branch of the right coronary artery is possible. To increase appreciably the stroke volume in cardiac tamponade at least 100 ml of blood should be aspirated. This may cause further fatal haemorrhage by raising the intracardiac pressure and disrupting the tamponade effect. Cardiac disruption caused by either blunt or penetrating trauma requires urgent surgical repair.

The plain chest radiograph

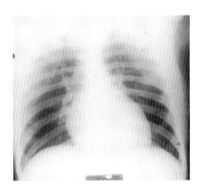

Cardiac tamponade caused by a left parasternal stab wound.

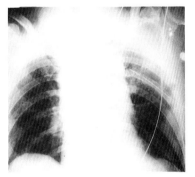

Aortic transection caused by a deceleration accident.

Plain chest radiography is the most important investigation in patients with thoracic trauma and should be undertaken with the patient erect or semi-erect if possible. This will enable the best assessment of the volume of free air or blood in the chest. In practice, patients with multiple injuries usually undergo radiography in a supine, semi-erect, or lateral decubitus position, with the x rays passing anteroposteriorly.

Most serious injuries, including cardiac tamponade, transected aorta, lacerated diaphragm, and major airways injury, can be diagnosed or ruled out on the basis of chest radiographs. Decide whether the radiological appearances are those expected from the physical signs and mechanism of injury. Are there unsuspected findings? Remember that in as many as 15 per cent of patients with fractured ribs, pulmonary contusion, and surgical emphysema but no pneumothorax the pleural cavity has been obliterated by previous pneumonic adhesions. Free air within the chest wall and haemopneumothorax usually indicate superficial pulmonary laceration by fractured ribs whereas air in the mediastinum (with or without pneumothorax), pneumopericardium, and air deep to the deep cervical fascia of the neck suggest tracheobronchial disruption. This is confirmed by bronchoscopy.

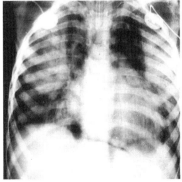

Free air in the mediastinum and beneath the deep cervical fascia owing to tracheal transection.

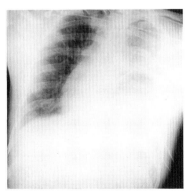

Ruptured left hemidiaphragm with haemothorax and stomach and ruptured spleen in left pleural cavity.

A widened mediastinum with associated features suggests rupture of the aorta and the need for control of blood pressure and early aortography. A fractured sternum or thoracic spine also causes widening of the mediastinum, as may arterial or venous injuries at the root of the neck. A widened mediastinum together with extrapleural apical capping in both hemithoraces strongly suggests aortic transection. Widening of the cardiac silhouette or an abnormal globular appearance of the heart suggests an intrapericardial haematoma. In association with clinical signs of cardiac tamponade this may need urgent pericardiocentesis or preferably median sternotomy or thoracotomy if cardiac disruption is suspected.

A lacerated left hemidiaphragm can normally be recognised by identifying bowel gas within the left hemithorax, usually in association with haemothorax. An apparent raised right hemidiaphragm suggests right diaphragmatic rupture as paralysis of the phrenic nerve caused by trauma is extremely rare. The possibility of a subdiaphragmatic haematoma from a ruptured liver can be excluded by abdominal ultrasonography.

In the absence of clinical or radiological evidence of major intrathoracic injury requiring early surgery treatment should be concentrated on moderating the pathophysiological processes that result from chest wall disruption, pulmonary contusion, and intrathoracic bleeding.

Radiological features that suggest aortic rupture

- Widening of the superior mediastinum to ≥8 cm in a 100 cm anteroposterior supine radiograph
- Tracheal shift to the right
- Blurring of the aortic outline
- Obliteration of the medial aspect of the left upper lobe (pleural capping)
- Opacification of the angle between the aorta and left pulmonary artery
- Depression of the left main bronchus to an angle <40° with the trachea

---

Chest drain insertion

One, and occasionally more than one, chest drain should be inserted to clear blood or air from the pleural cavity. Except under dire circumstances with tension pneumothorax a plain chest radiograph should be taken first. Surgical emphysema in the chest wall in the absence of a pneumothorax is not an indication for chest drain insertion, and drains should never be inserted prophylactically as damage to the underlying lung in patients with an obliterated pleural cavity may prove fatal.

In practice, drains are usually inserted for combined haemopneumothoraces. There are several simple steps to follow.

(1) Make certain that either blood or air is interposed between the chest wall and the lung. In about 15% of patients postpneumonic fibrous intrapleural adhesions obliterate the pleural space and result in the drain transfixing the lung

(2) Choose the site carefully: it will usually be between the fourth and seventh intercostal spaces, between the midaxillary and anterior axillary lines. The level at which the anterior axillary fold meets the chest wall is a useful guide. Consult the chest radiograph unless the drain is to be inserted as an absolute emergency. There is no contraindication to inserting the drain through an area of injury, but if there is possibility of a ruptured diaphragm with viscera in the chest the drain should be inserted high. Avoid the anterior approach in the second interspace as this transfixes the two major accessory respiratory muscles—the pectoralis major and minor. If an apical drain is required because of intrapleural adhesions towards the base then the true apical approach above the scapula and into the first interspace posteriorly is preferred. It is a fallacy that the drain must be in a basal position to drain blood and in an apical position to drain air.

(3) Choose a size >28 Argyle chest drain—smaller drains will rapidly occlude with blood clot. An established haemothorax will not drain and requires surgical evacuation.

(4) In conscious patients use between 10 and 15 ml of 1% lignocaine and infiltrate the periosteum on the upper border of the rib at the chosen interspace. Advancing the needle above the rib, the pleura should be infiltrated, and passage of the needle into the pleural cavity confirms the presence of free air or blood on aspiration. The needle can be left in situ so that the precise area of anaesthetic infiltration is not lost when the skin is cleansed with povidone-iodine solution.

(5) Use a scalpel to incise the chest wall about 2 cm beneath the proposed site of pleural incision, so that the drain track leads the drain to the apex of the pleural cavity. The scalpel should find the rib below the interspace to be breached, then the remainder of the track be completed through to the pleural cavity with artery forceps. This route avoids the intercostal nerve and, more importantly, the vessels that are protected underneath the ribs.

Chest drain insertion. (a) Penetration of the skin, muscle, and pleura. (b) Blunt dissection of the parietal pleura. (c) Exploration of the pleural cavities. (d) Tube directed posteriorly and superiorly.

The drain slides easily through the track and into the pleural cavity, when blood or air will flash-fill the tube. Do not be concerned about allowing air to enter along the drains; this will be evacuated immediately when the lung expands and there is underwater sealed drainage.

(6) When the drain is in position it is sutured with at least a zero gauge silk or propylene suture to prevent displacement. A pursestring suture is applied around the site.

(7) Always apply negative pressure to chest drains to ensure evacuation of continued haemorrhage or air leak. Never clamp the drain in the presence of a brisk air leak. A Thompson or Tubbs-Barrett suction machine is necessary to ensure large volume suction at a negative pressure of 15-20 cm H_2O. The Roberts suction pump should not be used as it will take only a small volume and may constitute an obstruction in the case of rapid air leak.

(8) Check the position and effect of the drain in a plain chest radiograph. Note the initial volume of blood evacuated and the continued rate of drainage on suction. Assess the volume of air leak. The need for thoracotomy is determined by the rate of bleeding or air leak through the drain during suction. In most patients the intercostal drain is the definitive intervention.

Chest wall derangement

Management of rib fractures

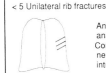

< 5 Unilateral rib fractures

Antipyretic oral or intravenous analgesia, physiotherapy
Consider local intercostal nerve block or intrapleural bupivacaine

Stable chest wall
Normal blood gas tensions

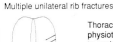

Multiple unilateral rib fractures

Thoracic epidural anaesthesia, physiotherapy, mini-tracheostomy to aspirate secretions
Consider surgical chest wall fixation

Stable or flail chest wall
Poor blood gas tensions

Transition depends on deterioration of blood gas tensions

Multiple fractures with deformity or bilateral fractures

Ventilation, physiotherapy
Consider surgical chest wall fixation and antibiotic prophylaxis

Unstable chest wall
Poor blood gas tensions

The two main types of serious chest wall derangement are a functionally important traumatic defect (sucking chest wound) and a flail segment. The most extensive disruption occurs in severe crush injuries in which multiple bilateral rib fractures and fractures of the sternum coexist. Each rib fracture is associated with a blood loss of about 150 ml. With multiple fractures blood loss may be substantial and is increased by laceration of the underlying lung by sharp edges. The damaged chest wall may be stable, so that with adequate pain relief breathing continues unhindered, or unstable, when the mechanics of breathing are compromised. The flail segment moves inwards on inspiration and consequently compromises ventilation by reducing tidal volume. Full expansion of the lung must be restored as soon as possible by covering a traumatic defect, stabilising a flail segment, and draining a haemopneumothorax. Further management is aimed not at the chest wall itself but at preserving respiratory function.

Pain causes decreased respiratory excursion and failure to ventilate the basal segments, resulting in atelectasis. Pain also inhibits cough so that secretions cannot be cleared from the bronchial tree, causing bronchial obstruction and acute respiratory failure. Pain relief is very important so that the most effective therapeutic option, physiotherapy, can be carried out frequently and with the patient's full cooperation.

Recent studies have shown decreased mortality in patients with extensive rib fractures with the conservative approach to pain relief compared with routine mechanical ventilation. This also applies to patients who have undergone surgery for concomitant abdominal or orthopaedic injuries, those with flail segments, and those with pulmonary or cardiac contusion as long as arterial Po_2 is >50 mm Hg when 50% oxygen is being inspired and vital capacity is >10 ml/kg. Analgesia is planned to provide a central block at the dermatome area of pain up to the level of T4. Intubation and ventilation should be considered only if the arterial Po_2 falls below 50 mm Hg with supplementary oxygen or if there is an increase in respiratory rate to 40 breaths/min with an inability to cough.

Mechanical ventilation is important in unconscious and uncooperative patients with severe or worsening respiratory failure despite adequate analgesia and clearance of secretions by physiotherapy. A flail segment in itself is not an indication for mechanical ventilation; the functional rather than the anatomical consequences of injury determine the necessity for ventilatory support. Surgical intervention is only rarely indicated for fixing sternal fractures, correcting serious deformities, and evacuating an extensive clotted haemothorax or haemostasis in a severely lacerated lung.

OTHER LIFE THREATENING CONDITIONS

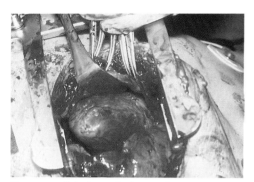

Exposure of the heart for immediate repair of a cardiac stab wound.

The plan of action in the treatment of patients with thoracic trauma depends on the initial findings on chest radiography, results of intercostal drainage, overall clinical state of the patient, and the relative priorities of associated visceral, vascular, and bony injuries.

Ruptured aorta

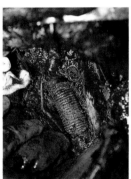

Traumatic transection of the thoracic aorta repaired by a Dacron tube graft.

The most common location of ruptured aorta is just distal to the origin of the subclavian artery and ligamentum arteriosum. The transection may be partial, complete, or spiral, and immediate survival depends on the formation of an acute false aneurysm. Diagnosis depends on a high index of suspicion then chest radiography followed by aortography.

An aortogram is always required as the sites of aortic injury may be multiple. The patient must be investigated in the hospital where surgery will be performed with the surgeon and team on site, as deterioration often follows injection of contrast fluid. If there is no thoracic surgeon the patient must be transferred to a cardiothoracic centre. Reliable blood pressure control must be maintained during transfer: patients with transected aorta are hypertensive owing to inappropriate baroreceptor responses and are therefore subject to exsanguination. It is best to transfer the patient intubated, ventilated, and heavily sedated or anaesthetised. On arrival at the cardiothoracic centre the department of radiology must be fully prepared.

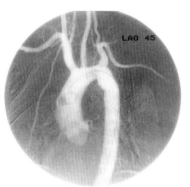

Aortogram showing laceration at the usual site after a deceleration injury.

If the angiogram confirms an aortic injury the treatment is by surgery and should take priority over all but immediately life threatening haemorrhage. During preparation for the operating theatre the patient's blood pressure is kept below 100 mm Hg with an infusion of sodium nitroprusside. Aortic repair is by direct suture of the laceration or by graft replacement of the injured area.

Blunt cardiac injury

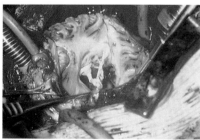

Lacerated tricuspid valve after a blunt cardiac injury. The valve was repaired on cardiopulmonary bypass.

Whereas a penetrating injury to the heart is usually obvious cardiac contusion is rarely considered before the onset of life threatening arrhythmia, cardiogenic shock, or cardiac arrest. Myocardial contusion occurs in patients with deceleration trauma and constitutes the most common unsuspected fatal injury. Two dimensional echocardiographic evidence of abnormal ventricular wall motion and pericardial effusion are the most reliable early clues to important myocardial damage. The possibility of blunt cardiac injury must be determined during resuscitation and assessed as soon as is practical as right ventricular dysfunction may demand higher filling pressures to maintain cardiac output.

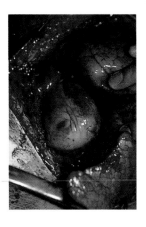

Immediate thoracotomy for blunt trauma with cardiac herniation. The severely contused heart was strangulated in the atrioventricular groove. The patient required an intra-aortic balloon pump for three days.

Myocardial contusion is roughly equivalent to acute myocardial infarction and should be treated appropriately. Cardiogenic shock is rarely seen with myocardial contusion alone, but adequate maintenance of perfusion pressure to uninjured cardiac muscle by using the intra-aortic balloon pump may be required.

Electrical instability at the sites of unevenly perfused myocardium initiates re-entry responses conducive to tachyarrhythmia. The electrocardiogram may show non-specific ST and T wave changes, sinus tachycardia, and conduction abnormalities such as right bundle branch block. Sudden death from complete heart block may occur early during convalescence, and persistent conduction defects may require a pacemaker. Acute or delayed cardiac rupture, ventricular septal rupture, and avulsion of the tricuspid and mitral valves may occur and require surgical correction by cardiopulmonary bypass.

Injury to major airways

Signs of injury to major airways

Free air
Subcutaneous or deep cervical emphysema
Pneumothorax
Pneumomediastinum
Pneumopericardium

Haemoptysis

Airways obstruction
Stridor
Aphonia
Difficult intubation

Extensive free air in the neck, mediastinum, or chest wall should always raise the suspicion of major airways injury. Transected trachea and bronchus proximal to the pleural reflection cause extensive mediastinal and deep cervical emphysema, which may spread to the subcutaneous tissues. Pneumothorax occurs when there is bronchial laceration distal to the pleural sheath. All levels of the trachea or main bronchi may be involved, though more than 80 per cent of injuries occur within 2·5 cm of the carina with equal distribution between right and left sides. The type of lesion varies from simple linear mucosal laceration to full thickness tears in the trachea, main bronchi, and branch bronchi.

The diagnosis is suggested by detection of free air on physical examination and chest radiography and confirmed by bronchoscopy. A rigid Negus or Stortz instrument is preferred as bronchoscopy must also clear the airway by removing blood clots and debris. The site, nature, and extent of injury are carefully defined. Torn bronchial mucosa and oedema may obscure the true extent of injury, and care must be taken not to displace the ends of a transected trachea or bronchus if a satisfactory airway exists. Treatment is usually by early primary repair, though conservative treatment is permissible if a longitudinal tear in the posterior tracheal membrane is short or if a bronchial tear is less than one third of the circumference and chest tube drainage fully re-expands the lung. Mini-tracheostomy can be performed to maintain a low intratracheal pressure and discourage leakage of air into the mediastinum while the mucosal laceration heals spontaneously.

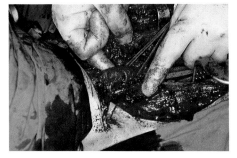

Stab wounds in the thoracic inlet. Exposure of the transected trachea and oesophagus by median sternotomy.

Lacerated diaphragm

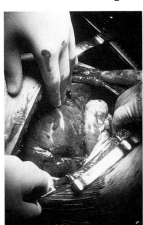

Ruptured left hemidiaphragm with the stomach in the chest.

Lacerated diaphragm is commonly overlooked if positive pressure ventilation, undertaken urgently, masks respiratory distress and signs such as bowel sounds in the left chest. Ventilation may also replace some of the viscera back into the abdomen and prevent gastric distension.

Ruptured left hemidiaphragm is more common as the right side is protected by the liver. Bilateral rupture is rare but can be encountered even in the absence of visceral injury. It is not unusual to overlook diaphragmatic rupture during laparotomy for hepatic or splenic rupture.

Surgical repair should be undertaken immediately unless exsanguinating haemorrhage or intracranial lesions take priority. If the tear is recognised early in a patient with abdominal injuries the transabdominal surgical approach is acceptable, though satisfactory access to the right hemidiaphragm is difficult. In the absence of intra-abdominal injury diaphragmatic repair is best undertaken by thoracotomy. When penetrating injuries pass through the diaphragm the defect should be closed to prevent strangulating hernia, particularly on the left side. However, not all patients with such injuries meet the criteria for thoracotomy or laparotomy.

The illustration of chest drain insertion was prepared by the department of education and medical illustration services, St Bartholomew's Hospital.

MANAGEMENT OF HYPOVOLAEMIC SHOCK

Peter J F Baskett

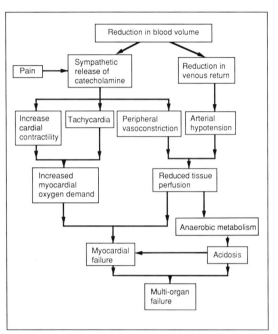

Pathophysiology of hypovolaemic shock.

Hypovolaemic shock is a clinical state in which tissue perfusion is rendered relatively inadequate by loss of blood or plasma after injury to the vascular tree.

A reduction in blood volume produces a fall in systolic pressure, which triggers a sympathetic catecholamine response that results in peripheral vasoconstriction, a rise in pulse rate, and a reduction in pulse pressure. The tachycardia and increased cardiac contractility lead to an increased myocardial oxygen requirement.

Blood flow to the skin and peripheral tissues is reduced in an effort to preserve reasonable perfusion of vital organs such as the brain, heart, liver, and kidneys. If there is continuing blood loss inadequate tissue perfusion results in anaerobic metabolism, acidosis, and reduction in the performance of the vital organs. Further myocardial depression accelerates this process, and pain stimuli add to the sympathetic outburst.

Classification of hypovolaemic shock according to blood loss

	Class I	Class II	Class III	Class IV
Blood loss:				
Percentage	<15	15-30	30-40	>40
Volume (ml)	750	800-1500	1500-2000	>2000
Blood pressure:				
Systolic	Unchanged	Normal	Reduced	Very low
Diastolic	Unchanged	Raised	Reduced	Very low or unrecordable
Pulse (beats/min)	Slight tachycardia	100-120	120 (Thready)	>120 (Very thready)
Capillary refill	Normal	Slow (>2s)	Slow (>2s)	Undetectable
Respiratory rate	Normal	Normal	Tachypnoea (>20/min)	Tachypnoea (>20/min)
Urinary flow rate (ml/h)	>30	20-30	10-20	0-10
Extremities	Colour normal	Pale	Pale	Pale and cold
Complexion	Normal	Pale	Pale	Ashen
Mental state	Alert	Anxious or agressive	Anxious, agressive, or drowsy	Drowsy, confused, or unconscious

Symptoms of hypovolaemia according to blood loss

Blood loss (ml)	Class	Symptoms
<750	I	None
−1500	II	Cardiovascular signs due to catecholamine release: thirst, weakness, tachypnoea
−2000	III	Systolic pressure falls
>2000	IV	Systolic pressure becomes unreadable

The following are early symptoms and signs of hypovolaemic shock. They reflect the underlying pathophysiology.

- Hypotension (due to hypovolaemia, perhaps followed by myocardial insufficiency)
- Skin pallor (vasoconstriction due to catecholamine release)
- Tachycardia (due to catecholamine release)
- Confusion, aggression, drowsiness, and coma (due to cerebral hypoxia and acidosis)
- Tachypnoea (due to hypoxia and acidosis)
- General weakness (due to hypoxia and acidosis)
- Thirst (due to hypovolaemia)
- Reduced urine output (due to reduced perfusion).

In most cases the signs and symptoms can be related to the amount of blood loss, which can be classified in four broad groups (classes I-IV).

In previously healthy young adults systolic pressure is often preserved despite quite appreciable blood loss (1·5-2·0 litres) owing to the effective response to sympathetic stimulation. Eventually, however, there is a precipitous fall as the myocardium suddenly fails because of hypoxia and acidosis. Conversely, patients with coronary arterial disease may become hypotensive because of myocardial insufficiency after only modest blood losses of up to 500 ml.

Patients receiving certain drugs (for example, β blockers) may not be able to produce an appropriate sympathetic response and may also become hypotensive after modest blood loss. Also, it must be taken into account that intravascular loss is accompanied by additional fluid depletion of the interstitial space, which amounts to about 25% of the overt blood loss.

Resuscitation of patients with trauma
(1) Adequate pulmonary oxygenation
(2) Control of haemorrhage
(3) Replacement of lost volume
(4) Monitoring the effects of (1), (2), and (3)
(5) Support of myocardial contractility
(6) Relief of pain

Generally, losses of up to 750 ml (class I) (15% of the circulating blood volume) do not generate any pronounced signs or symptoms. Further haemorrhage, amounting to 1·5 litres (class II), produces cardiovascular signs of catecholamine release, thirst, weakness, and tachypnoea. Systolic pressure continues to fall as blood loss mounts to 2 litres (class III) and often becomes unreadable after 2·5-3·0 litres (class IV) have been lost.

The objective of the management of hypovolaemic shock is to maintain tissue oxygenation and restore it to normal values. This entails applying the basic principles of resuscitation of patients with trauma. Resuscitation is followed by definitive treatment (including surgery).

Pulmonary oxygenation

Ventilate patients with hypovolaemic shock
Use 100% oxygen for patients with severe shock

To ensure optimal pulmonary oxygenation patients with hypovolaemic shock should have a clear airway and be adequately ventilated with oxygen at a high inspired concentration. Unconscious patients with severe shock should be intubated and ventilated with 100% oxygen, and care should be taken to exclude impairment of ventilation due to pneumothorax, haemothorax, or diaphragmatic elevation caused by gastric distention.

Control of haemorrhage

For peripheral haemorrhage: "Parts in the air, press on the hole"

Peripheral haemorrhage should be controlled by elevation of the injured part and by placing a firm pad and bandage over the wound. Tourniquets are rarely advised though may be essential and are relatively harmless in patients who are going to undergo amputation. Probing in the wound to search for ruptured vessels is not recommended outside the operating room.

Replacement of loss

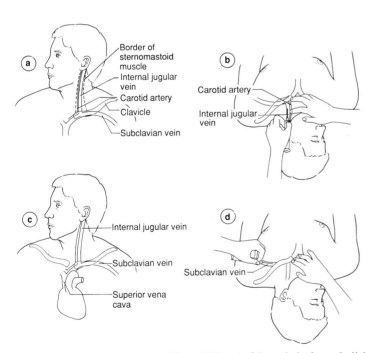

Cannulation of the jugular vein ((a) and (b)) and of the subclavian vein ((c) and (d)).

Losses of blood should be replaced intravenously in response to clinical signs and symptoms and in all patients estimated to have lost more than 750 ml.

Intravenous cannulation

The site of haemorrhage should be considered carefully when cannulation is undertaken. There is little point in setting up an infusion in an injured limb or in the femoral vein in a patient with pelvic or abdominal injuries. With this proviso the peripheral veins of the arm, if accessible, are traditionally preferred for cannulation. There is much to be said, however, for more central access through a short cannula in the subclavian or internal jugular vessels, which are less subject to constriction and feed almost directly into the right atrium. Preference for one or other site is individual according to experience and expertise. In patients with injuries of the neck and arms the femoral vein is preferable. Venous cut down techniques are time consuming, rarely necessary, and usually less effective than direct cannulation of a central vein.

The diameter of the cannula in a cannula over needle system should be not less than 14 gauge. Cannulas of 10 gauge can be easily inserted into the internal jugular or subclavian veins. Long lines from the antecubital fossa are not suitable for rapid transfusion as the flow rate is inversely related to the length of the catheter.

Management of hypovolaemic shock

<table>
<tr><td colspan="2">Intravenous fluid replacement in haemorrhagic shock</td></tr>
<tr><td>Class I
(haemorrhage
750 ml (15%))</td><td>2·5 l Ringer-lactate
solution or 1·0 l
polygelatin</td></tr>
<tr><td>Class II
(haemorrhage 800
-1500 ml (15-30%))</td><td>1·0 l polygelatin plus 1·5 l
Ringer-lactate solution</td></tr>
<tr><td>Class III
(haemorrhage
1500-2000 ml (30-
40%))</td><td>1·0 l Ringer-lactate
solution plus 0·5 l
polygelatin plus 1·0-1·5 l
whole blood or 1·0-1·5 l
equal volumes of
concentrated red cells
and polygelatin</td></tr>
<tr><td>Class IV
(haemorrhage
2000 ml (48%))</td><td>1·0 l Ringer-lactate
solution plus 1·0 l
polygelatin plus 2·0 l
whole blood or 2·0 l equal
volumes concentrated
red cells and polygelatin
or hetastarch</td></tr>
</table>

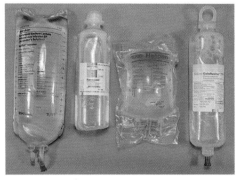

Intravenous replacement fluids.

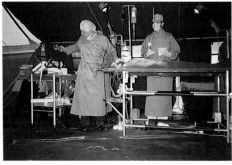

Intravenous infusion in a military surgery.

Disadvantages of blood transfusion in hypovolaemic shock

- Time is required to group and cross match individual units of blood

- Blood has a high viscosity and the microcirculation in shock may be improved by a reduction in packed cell volume

- Blood stored for more than a few days has a high potassium ion concentration and the platelets and white cells fragment rapidly, losing normal function

- Blood and certain blood products may be infected. (The risk of acquiring HIV infection from transfused blood has been virtually eliminated in the United Kingdom)

Choice of intravenous fluid

Intravenous fluids should be given to restore an adequate circulating blood volume. Normal electrolyte and coagulation constituents and colloid osmotic pressure and a packed cell volume above 30% are necessary to ensure adequate oxygen carrying capacity. The choice of intravenous fluids in clinical practice lies among crystalloid, colloid, and albumin solutions; blood in the form of whole blood or packed red cells; and a judicious mix of all of these.

Colloid solutions replace intravascular loss and restore haemodynamic values towards normal. They do not replace interstitial loss. Crystalloid solutions replace both interstitial and intravascular loss, but large volumes are required to restore normal haemodynamics. In practice, a combination of a crystalloid solution and a colloid solution should be given to patients with blood loss of more than 1 litre.

Colloid solutions are generally iso-oncotic and may be used to replace lost volumes of blood on a 1:1 basis, restoring haemodynamic variables to normal values. Polygelatins are cheap and effective blood volume expanders. They have a long shelf life of six years, a half life in vivo of six to eight hours, and a low index of causing anaphylatic reactions. Haemaccel has a similar electrolyte content to plasma whereas Gelofusine contains very little potassium. Both are suitable for replacing blood losses of up to 1 litre and in patients with more extensive haemorrhage when used in combination with blood transfusion to maintain a packed cell volume of 30%.

Hetastarch (6% in isotonic saline) is an effective blood substitute in patients with mild and moderate blood loss. It is more expensive than the polygelatins but has a much longer half life (12 to 14 hours) in the circulation. Care must be taken, therefore, to avoid circulation overload when blood is transfused at a later stage to restore the packed cell volume. The incidence of anaphylactic reactions is low.

Crystalloid solutions—Ringer-lactate solution may be used in patients with mild class I haemorrhage of up to 15% of blood volume. Replacement volumes should be three to four times the estimated loss as the electrolyte solution is distributed throughout the extracellular (intravascular and interstitial) space. The volume should be increased to compensate for urine loss. Vascular support with isotonic electrolyte solutions is short lived.

Blood—Whole blood or packed red cells are required in patients with moderate and major blood loss to maintain a packed cell volume of 30%. It is not desirable to strive for higher values in the early stages of volume resuscitation as a modest reduction in packed cell volume allows improvement in the microcirculation, especially in the presence of arteriolar vasoconstriction.

Though whole blood is the ideal replacement in patients with major haemorrhage, limitations of supply may dictate that concentrated red cells are used, diluted to normal values of packed cell volume by concurrent transfusion of polygelatin or hetastarch.

Trauma and obstetric centres should retain a small number of relatively fresh units of O negative blood for immediate transfusion in cases of severe, life threatening haemorrhage.

Blood transfused rapidly should be warmed before infusion to maximise flow rates and to minimise the risk of cardiac arrhythmia and core hypothermia. Blood filters have not been proved to be of value.

Autologous blood—In patients with severe thoracic or abdominal injuries "clean" blood may be aspirated from the cavity, anticoagulated, and returned to the patient through an intravenous cannula using a "cell saver" system. Autologous blood is valuable in patients with major vascular injuries of the thorax and abdomen and in those with a ruptured liver or spleen, but clearly the procedure cannot be applied in patients with abdominal trauma who have a ruptured bowel or in those with thoracic trauma who have oesophageal or lung damage. The transfusion of autologous blood has several advantages, particularly if blood of a patient's blood group is in short supply. The blood is the patient's own, free of infection, warm, and immediately available.

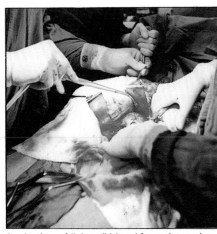

Aspiration of "clean" blood from the cavity.

Coagulation problems

Coagulation problems occur in patients with massive blood loss because of dilution with blood substitutes and the fact that coagulation factors deteriorate rapidly in stored blood. Moreover, tissue destruction releases various products that inhibit the normal coagulation process. The clotting process should be monitored by regular screening and deficiencies treated definitively rather than by infusion of valuable fresh frozen plasma and platelets on an arbitrary basis.

Monitoring progress and treatment

Variables to monitor
• Pulse rate
• Arterial pressure
• Pulse pressure
• Central venous pressure
• Urinary output
• Changes in the electrocardiogram
• Temperature
• Peripheral oxygen saturation
• End tidal carbon dioxide levels
• Mental state

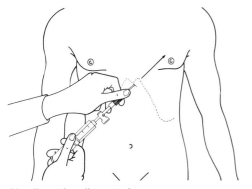

Needle pericardiocentesis.

Requirements for blood volume replacement should be based on all of factors in the box, particularly pulse rate, arterial pulse and central venous pressures, peripheral oxygen saturation, and urine flow rates. Transfusion should be continued to produce an adequate arterial pressure, a urine flow of 50 ml/h, and a central venous pressure that responds to a rapid infusion of 200 ml by a sustained rise of more than 3 cm H_2O over the previous value.

If these variables improve and the improvement is maintained then clearly the blood loss is under control. Failure to maintain the improved values indicates continuing loss and requires further transfusion and early surgery. If the patient does not respond satisfactorily to transfusions the rate of loss is exceeding the fastest possible rate of intravenous replacement. This is usually associated with major thoracic, abdominal, or pelvic injuries. In such instances the patient must be taken to the operating room for immediate thoracotomy or laparotomy and bleeding controlled with clamps or packs, or both, while the anaesthetist "catches up" with the transfusion requirements. Salvage of autologous blood may be appropriate.

A rising central venous pressure associated with a low arterial pressure, tachycardia, and a reduced urine output indicates tension pneumothorax, cardiac tamponade, or cardiac failure. Cardiac tamponade is treated by thoracotomy, sometimes preceded by relief needle paracentesis. In patients requiring inotropic support because of myocardial failure measurement of pulmonary wedge pressure and cardiac output with a Swan-Ganz catheter or non-invasive method may be helpful in comparing individual ventricular load and performance. In most patients with previously normal hearts, however, the central venous pressure and the pulmonary artery wedge pressure follow each other closely and the extra expense of this invasive technique is unjustified.

Maintenance of normal carbon dioxide and oxygen tensions will optimise cerebral perfusion.

Cardiac contractility and renal output

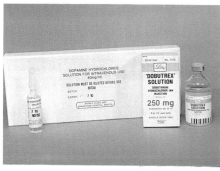

Inotropic drugs.

A patient with a previously impaired myocardium may need inotropic support with dopamine and dobutamine. Such support is not a substitute for adequate volume replacement but is used to enhance myocardial contraction if required. Rates of dopamine infusion should be confined to "renal" doses (up to 5 µg/kg/h) that enhance urine output. Higher doses cause vasoconstriction and tachycardia, which results in an increase in myocardial oxygen demand that may not be achievable because of inadequate myocardial blood flow. Dobutamine should than be added to improve myocardial performance.

Pain relief

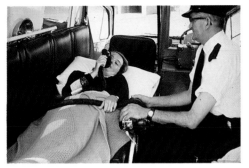

Patient receiving Entonox on the way to hospital.

Pain relief must be given not only for its compassionate value but also for its essential beneficial influence on the pathophysiology of hypovolaemic shock in reducing catecholamine secretion. Giving a mixture of 50% nitrous oxide and 50% oxygen (Entonox) is of value before the patient reaches hospital, and this should be supplemented with increments of intravenous morphine 5 mg, nalbuphine 10 mg, or ketamine 25-50 mg with diazepam 5-10 mg or midazolam 5 mg until analgesia is achieved.

Conclusion

The photograph showing aspiration of blood was reproduced by kind permission of Solco Basle. The line drawings were prepared by the department of education and medical illustration services, St Bartholomew's Hospital.

Many patients will die of hypovolaemic shock despite the fact that the principles of management and treatment should be well known and understood. Too often, however, in retrospect the treatment offered was too little, too late, allowing a malignant circle of pathophysiological changes to be irreversibly established. Early aggressive treatment offers the best results.

Pneumatic counter pressure suit

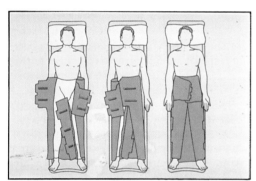

Pneumatic counter pressure suit.

Pneumatic counter pressure suits (medical anti-shock trousers) have been used extensively, particularly in the United States, to control haemorrhage from the legs, pelvis, and abdomen and spinal shock. The suit consists of inflatable sections for each leg and the abdomen and is radiotranslucent with access for urinary catheterisation and digital rectal examination.

Application of the suit produces:
- Autotransfusion of 0·5-1·0 litres of homologous blood
- Reduction in haemorrhage from tissues beneath the suit
- Reduction in the total functioning volume of the vascular compartment, permitting relatively improved perfusion of the heart, brain, and arms (thereby assisting with intravenous cannulation)
- Splinting of limb and pelvic fractures with consequent reduction in blood loss and pain.

- Do not apply the abdominal section in pregnant women or patients with abdominal injury with protruding viscera
- Do not deflate the suit until at least two wide bore intravenous cannulas are safely in situ and an adequate supply of blood and blood substitute are available
- In patients with abdominal injuries or ruptured aortic aneurysm the suit should not be deflated until the patient is in the operating room and the surgical team ready to control haemorrhage
- Do not leave the suit inflated for more than one to two hours as ischaemic anaerobic metabolism may lead to profound general metabolic acidosis
- Take care not to overtransfuse patients with poor left ventricular function with the suit inflated because pulmonary oedema may occur.

The suit should be applied in patients with symptoms of hypovolaemia and a systolic blood pressure <90 mm Hg. Suit inflation pressures of 40-50 mm Hg (5·5-6·5 kPa) should be used initially, increasing to 80 mm Hg (10·5 kPa) if the systolic pressure does not improve. The time of application should be noted.

HEAD INJURIES

Ross Bullock, Graham Teasdale

Characteristics of patients with head injuries attending accident and emergency departments in Scotland. Numbers are percentages of patients

Male	70
Adult	60
Recently drunk alcohol	25
Type of injury:	
Scalp laceration	40
Skull fracture	2
Conscious level:	
Never unconscious	80
Recovered from amnesia	15
Impaired	3·5
Cause of injury:	
Fall	14
Assault	16
Road traffic accident	18
Domestic	18
Sport	12
Work	8

Staff in an accident and emergency department serving a population of 250 000 people can expect to treat about 5000 patients each year who have suffered a head injury—10% of their work. Most attenders are only mildly injured, but head injuries have a reputation for being treacherous. A traumatic intracranial haematoma will develop in fewer than 12 patients each year but can transform an initially mild injury into a life threatening emergency. In the small number of patients (less than 5%) who present with persistent impaired consciousness correct diagnosis and assignment of priorities can be life saving. The limited availability of specialist neurosurgical facilities in the United Kingdom means that doctors can admit only 1% of the patients who attend with head injuries.

Role of accident and emergency department in management of head injuries

- Resuscitate, diagnose, and record
- Detect or exclude other injuries
- Request, supervise, and interpret results of radiography and other initial investigations
- Decide if admission is needed and if so, where
- Liaise with other specialties—for example, neurosurgery—about serious cases
- Ensure adequate arrangements for observing and maintaining patient's condition during transfer to other departments or hospitals
- Observe progress of patients with minor injuries, who should be admitted to short stay beds
- Ensure adequate arrangements for follow up

In recent years the task for staff in accident and emergency departments has been simplified by the development of agreed guidelines for management, thus reflecting the increased knowledge of the mechanisms of head injury, improved methods of assessment and diagnosis, and more accurate identification of patients at risk of brain damage.

The two main aims of management of patients with head injuries are, firstly, to provide the best conditions for recovery from any brain damage already sustained and, secondly, to prevent or treat complications leading to secondary brain damage.

Mechanisms of brain damage

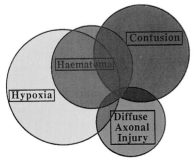

Causes of brain damage after severe head injury.

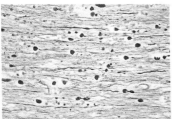

Retraction balls—the microscopic feature of diffuse axonal injury.

Diffuse damage

The brain is poorly anchored within the skull and its soft consistency renders it liable to move within the skull in response to acceleration or deceleration.

Contact between the surface of the brain and the interior skull causes bruising (contusions), particularly at the frontal and temporal poles. Distortion of the brain caused by internal shearing forces leads to stretching and tearing of axonal tracts within the white matter. Such diffuse axonal injury manifests itself as microscopic retraction balls at the site of damaged fibres; these are widespread in severe injuries, but mild stretch injury with reversible loss of function is also responsible for the transient disturbance of consciousness known as "concussion."

Head injuries

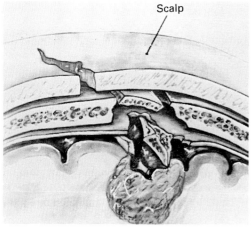

Scalp

Compound depressed skull fracture.

Focal impact damage

Skull fracture—At the point of impact the skull deforms inwards and a fracture may occur. Such fractures are less common in children than in adults because of their more elastic skulls.

A compound depressed fracture results when a violent sharp blow lacerates the scalp and drives bone fragments into the intracranial cavity, sometimes tearing the dura mater. This injury is an important source of intracranial infection and requires prompt surgical elevation and debridement. A depressed fracture is also a powerful cause of epilepsy, but the risk of this complication is not influenced by surgical treatment.

A linear fracture is important chiefly as an indicator of secondary intracranial bleeding.

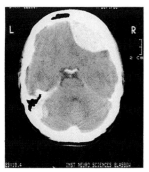

Moderate sized right frontal extradural haematoma.

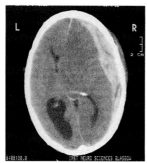

Large right subdural haematoma with pronounced midline shift and contralateral ventricular dilatation.

Extradural haematoma—The inbending of the skull may strip off underlying dura and create a space in which an extradural haematoma develops. This can be associated with little primary brain damage, and optimal management should minimise mortality and morbidity due to secondary cerebral compression. Delayed treatment can cause irreversible cerebral damage.

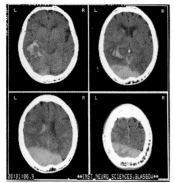

Large occipital extradural haematoma overlying confluence of intracranial venous sinuses with left temporal contusion.

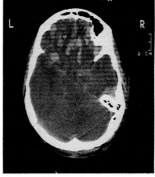

Multiple bifrontal cerebral contusion caused by a fall on to the occiput (a "contra-coup" injury).

Intradural haematoma—Subdural and intracerebral bleeding are four times more common than extradural haematoma. They result from tearing of cerebral veins or from laceration of the brain's surface, or both. An association with primary brain damage is common, but the outcome may nevertheless be good if an operation is performed promptly.

Hypoxia and ischaemia

The brain requires continuous perfusion with well oxygenated blood. Permanent ischaemic neuronal damage occurs if this is reduced below a critical threshold for more than a few minutes. Normally the brain regulates its own blood supply to maintain constant perfusion despite wide variations in systemic blood pressure; when injured, the brain loses this capacity and is thus particularly vulnerable to ischaemic damage when hypotension or hypoxia occur.

A reduction in mean arterial blood pressure to below 60-80 mm Hg, particularly when intracranial pressure is raised, may cause ischaemic neuronal damage if sustained for more than a few minutes. Multiply injured patients may become severely shocked immediately after injury.

When a head injury is severe enough to produce unconsciousness early respiratory disorders and bradycardia occur and are a potent cause of ischaemic damage. The airway is often compromised immediately after injury owing to mechanical obstruction or loss of protective reflexes.

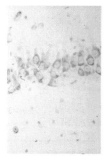 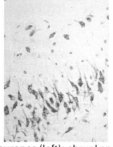

Normal hippocampal neurones (left); shrunken, pyknotic hippocampal neurones irreversibly damaged by ischaemia or hypoxia (right).

Causes of raised intracranial pressure after head injury

- Haematoma
- Focal cerebral oedema related to a contusion or haematoma
- Diffuse oedema after ischaemia (cytotoxic)
- Diffuse brain swelling ("brain engorgement")
- Obstruction of cerebrospinal fluid pathway (this is rare)

Raised intracranial pressure

About 70% of patients persistently in coma after severe head injury have raised intracranial pressure. This jeopardises cerebral perfusion because cerebral perfusion pressure is equal to mean arterial blood pressure minus intracranial pressure.

As intracranial pressure rises cerebrospinal fluid is driven out of the intracranial compartment—the first stage in compensation. As the pressure continues to rise brain shifts occur within the cranial cavity.

The most important of these brain shifts is uncal transtentorial herniation or "coning." This causes impairment of conscious level, development of a fixed dilated pupil, and brain stem compression with cardiovascular and respiratory abnormalities.

Intracranial contents within closed skull show shifts in response to haematoma.

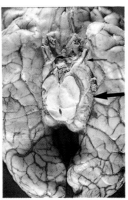

Midbrain sectioned at level of third cranial nerves shows uncal transtentorial herniation or "coning." Note bilateral "notching" of third nerves due to compression against tentorium.

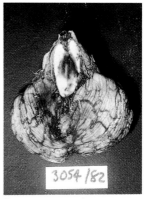

Consequences of unrelieved brainstem compression: "flame shaped" brainstem haemorrhage with irreversible damage to vital centres.

Management of head injuries

Glasgow coma chart.

For patients with a depressed conscious level the first priority is to stabilise circulation and respiration and prevent further secondary cerebral damage. The risks of secondary complications then need to be assessed and a decision made regarding transfer to a neurosurgical centre.

Additional factors

In addition to the factors recorded on the Glasgow coma chart the following should be recorded:

- Pupil diameter and reaction to light
- Pulse and blood pressure
- Temperature and respiration
- Movement of all limbs

All patients require ongoing recording of conscious level (by the Glasgow coma scale)—the best motor response should be used. To exclude traumatic tetraplegia the response to painful stimuli should be tested by supraorbital nerve compression if limb responses are absent. Patients observed may be either in hospital or, in certain cases, at home, provided that the patient can be discharged into the care of a responsible adult.

Head injuries

Management of patients who cannot talk

- **A**irway with cervical spine control—Definitive control of airway; keep a rigid cervical collar on
- **B**reathing—Analysis of blood gas tensions (Po$_2$>13 kPa (100 mm Hg) and Pco$_2$ <5·3 kPa (40 mm Hg) is acceptable)
- **C**irculation—If mean arterial blood pressure is <80 mm Hg infuse Hartmann's or Ringer solution or plasma until it is corrected
- **D**ysfunction of central nervous system— Check score on coma scale, pupils, limb movements
- **E**xposure and radiographs—Remove all clothing and examine "head to toe" (as described in the chapter on initial assessment). Obtain skull, chest, and cervical spine radiographs rapidly and ensure that the C7 vertebra is imaged

Priorities for management depend on whether the patient can talk. If he or she cannot do so both intracranial and extracranial complications are more likely.

In patients who can talk, document their history, duration of amnesia after trauma, mechanism of injury, previous medical and surgical history, and previous intake of drugs and alcohol.

In all cases after the secondary survey has been completed give prophylactic antibiotics for leakage of cerebrospinal fluid, basal skull fracture, compound fracture, or depressed fracture—for example, give penicillin two million units intravenously six hourly for seven days or orally as appropriate or co-trimoxazole 960 mg twice daily for seven days orally.

Indications for endotracheal intubation in patients with severe head injuries

- Absent gag reflex when oropharyngeal suction is attempted in unconscious patients
- When airway protection is needed—for example, when there is oropharyngeal bleeding, facial fracture, or vomitus that cannot be easily cleared by the patient
- When ventilation or blood gas tensions, or both, are too poor to allow spontaneous ventilation. (P$_a$O$_2$ <9 kPa breathing air or <13 kPa when receiving supplemental oxygen; P$_a$CO$_2$ >5·3 kPa.) (Exclude pneumothorax on the basis of the chest radiograph)
- To allow hyperventilation when a patient's condition is deteriorating because of raised intracranial pressure (after discussion with a neurosurgeon)

Guidelines for endotracheal intubation

If injury of the cervical spine has not been excluded intubate the patient with the neck stabilised by an assistant or by using sandbags. A full stomach should always be assumed and a rapid sequence of induction employed, with cricoid compression. Not all intubated patients require artificial ventilation.

Short acting drugs (for example, thiopentone, etomidate, propofol, and suxamethonium, atracurium, and vecuronium) should be used to facilitate intubation, which should be performed by an experienced person (usually an anaesthetist).

A cuffed endotracheal tube should be used, except in young children, and securely fixed to the patient with a neck halter and adhesive strapping. After intubation adjust the position of the tube to ensure that air entry is present in both lungs as intubation of the right main bronchus is common. An anaesthetist (or other experienced person) should accompany an intubated patient during transfer within the hospital or between hospitals.

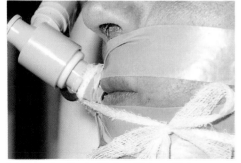

Intubated patient with head injury. Note secure fixation of endotracheal tube.

Indicators for skull radiography

If any of the following are present skull radiography should be performed:
- Neurological symptoms and signs
- Cerebrospinal fluid or blood from the nose or ear
- Suspected penetrating injury (it may be necessary to shave the hair)
- Pronounced bruising or swelling of the scalp.

Hospital admission

The following list of indications for admission of patients with head injuries should be displayed in accident and emergency departments.

- Confusion or any other depression of consciousness at the time of the examination
- Skull fracture
- Neurological symptoms or signs, or both
- Difficulty in assessing the patient—for example, because of ingestion of alcohol, epilepsy, or other medical conditions that cloud consciousness; children are also difficult to assess
- Lack of a responsible adult to supervise the patient and other social problems.

Brief amnesia after trauma with full recovery is not necessarily an indication for admission.

If the patient is to be observed outside hospital he or she should be discharged with a head injury "warning card" into the care of a responsible person.

The aims of hospital admission are to provide optimal conditions for recovery of the brain and to detect complications before they cause further secondary brain damage. The mainstay of admission is therefore neurological observation, which should be hourly for at least the first 24 hours.

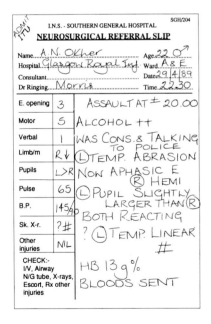

Consultation with a neurosurgeon

A group of British neurosurgeons formulated the following list of indications for consultation with a neurosurgeon and computed tomography in patients with head injuries.

(1) Fractured skull with confusion or worse impairment of consciousness, focal neurological signs, fits, or any other neurological symptoms or signs.

(2) Coma continuing after resuscitation, even if there is no skull fracture (coma is defined as not obeying commands, not speaking, not opening eyes—that is, a Glasgow coma score $\leqslant 8$).

(3) Deterioration in level of consciousness or development of other neurological signs.

(4) Confusion or other neurological disturbance persisting for more than six to eight hours even without skull fracture.

(5) Compound depressed fractures of the vault of the skull.

(6) Suspected fracture of the base of the skull—causing leakage of cerebrospinal fluid, orbital haematoma, or retromastoid haematoma—or other penetrating injury (for example, gunshot wounds).

Patients in categories 1-3 should be referred urgently. In all cases the diagnosis and initial treatment of serious extracranial injury takes priority over transfer to the nearest neurosurgical unit.

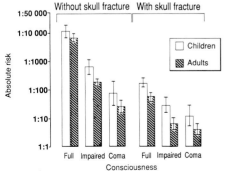

Absolute risk of intracranial haematoma in patients with head injury.

Computed tomography

Increasing numbers of accident and emergency departments have access to emergency computed tomography for patients with head injuries, but the interpretation of the computed tomogram is often difficult—for example, features of raised intracranial pressure can be missed by the untrained observer. It is preferable for computed tomography to be performed under the control of a neurosurgeon or neuroradiologist.

Drugs in acute head injury

Antibiotics in head injury

Indications

Basal fracture
Compound vault fracture
Suspected or proven meningitis

Suitable agents

Benzylpenicillin 1 million units intravenously every six hours for seven days or phenoxymethylpenicillin orally 500 mg every six hours (children 10-20 mg/kg/day)

For patients with penicillin allergy give oral co-trimoxazole 960 mg twice daily

---

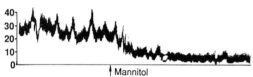

The effect of mannitol in a patient with raised intracranial pressure after severe focal brain injury.

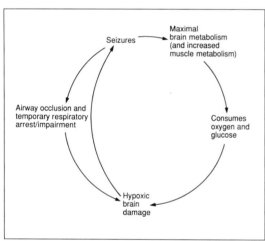

The consequences of uncontrolled seizures.

Sedation and analgesia

Sedation and analgesia for patients with head injuries are often a problem; they may be in pain and nauseous as a result of their injury, yet strong opiate analgesics and drugs with respiratory depressant effects must be avoided as they may cause iatrogenic deterioration in conscious level and respiratory depression. For adults give paracetamol 250-500 mg every six hours or dihydrocodeine preparations such as DF118, or Co-codamol one to two tablets every four to six hours. If given parenterally DF118, 30 mg every six hours is usually safe and effective. Give metoclopramide 10 mg up to every eight hours for nausea intravenously or orally. For children paracetamol suspension 125-250 mg every six hours is suitable.

Antibiotics

Avoid using antibiotics prophylactically except in the cases described in the box.

Mannitol

Mannitol is a powerful osmotic diuretic and may be life saving, but it carries dangers. It should be used, in consultation with a neurosurgeon, to "buy time" while the patient is prepared for transfer to the nearest neurosurgical centre. Give 0·5-1 g/kg as a bolus over 10-30 minutes. (Usually 250-400 ml of a 20% solution for adults.)

Steroids

Several trials have shown no benefit from steroids, even at high doses.

Management of seizures

Seizures within the first week carry a low risk of future epilepsy but may cause severe hypoxic brain damage. Prevent further seizures with phenytoin as a loading dose of a 250 mg bolus given intravenously over 10 minutes (ideally with electrocardiography) followed by an intravenous infusion of 250-500 mg over four hours. Thereafter give 100 mg every eight hours intravenously or orally.

If seizures persist after phenytoin loading give clonazepam 0·25 mg intravenously incrementally after each seizure. Be prepared to ventilate the patient in an intensive care unit. Intravenous diazepam 5-10 mg may be used if seizures still persist but may cause respiratory depression.

Restlessness

In patients with head injury restlessness is often a warning sign, and restless patients should not be sedated without excluding hypoxia, hypotension, metabolic derangement, a full bladder, or pain due to other injuries. The "checklist" for secondary deterioration described below should be considered before sedation is prescribed.

Secondary deterioration in conscious level

Effect of hypotension and hypoxia on patients' outcome after acute head injury

	Outcome	
	Dead/ vegetative/ severely disabled	Moderate disability, good recovery
Both hypoxia and hypotension	6	
Hypoxia only	11	7
Hypotension only	1	1
Neither hypoxia nor hypotension	11	38

$\chi^2 = 14·72$; $p < 0·005$.

If deterioration in conscious level is apparent the following possibilities should be investigated.

Hypoxia—Check arterial blood gas tensions, respiratory rate, and chest radiographs. Start treatment with oxygen.

Ischaemia—Check pulse, blood pressure, electrocardiogram, and full blood count, particularly if there has been a substantial delay between the patient sustaining the head injury and assessment. Exclude intra-abdominal bleeding.

Metabolic derangement—Exclude dehydration and check urea, electrolyte, and blood glucose concentrations.

Missed intracranial haematoma—If hypoxia, ischaemia, and metabolic derangement have been excluded refer the patient for computed tomography.

Seizures—Seizures may not have been witnessed. Control them with drugs. If the conscious level has not returned to its previous level within one hour consult the neurosurgeon.

Guide to siting of exploratory burr holes

(1) Give 0·5 g/kg of 20% mannitol solution intravenously over 15 minutes while the theatre is prepared

(2) Perform the procedure with the patient intubated and under general anaesthesia. Blood should be cross matched and an intravenous line (preferably plus a central venous line) established

(3) Shave, prepare, and drape the patient for "whole head" access

(4) Place the first burr hole adjacent to the fracture, ipsilateral to the first pupil to dilate or, in the absence of a fracture, in the temporal region (2·5 cm above the zygoma and 2·5 cm behind the zygomaticofrontal ridge)

(5) If an extradural clot is found enlarge the hole, following the clot

(6) If the underlying dura is blue and tense enlarge the burr hole to 5-8 cm in diameter and open the dura and evacuate as much clot as possible. Seek neurosurgical advice

(7) If no clot is seen beneath the dura make frontal and parietal burr holes ipsilateral to the first dilated pupil

(8) If no haematoma is found needling the brain is unlikely to be useful. Close the burr holes and refer the patient to the neurosurgical centre

Meningitis—If meningitis is suspected first obtain a computed tomogram to exclude the presence of a haematoma, which may cause neck stiffness. Start treatment with high doses of antibiotics immediately. Lumbar puncture should be performed only after computed tomography has excluded raised intracranial pressure. (Appropriate antibiotic treatment is intravenous penicillin 5 million units every six hours and intravenous chloramphenicol 1-2 g every six hours.)

Exploratory burr holes

The use of exploratory burr holes in modern management of head injury is extremely limited. Even experienced neurosurgeons miss one third of intracranial haematomas and may initiate bleeding and worsen brain damage. Use of burr holes may be indicated if a capable surgeon is available and a previously alert patient rapidly deteriorates and develops a fixed dilated pupil that is ipsilateral to a skull fracture and in patients whose transfer to a neurosurgical centre is likely to take two hours or more.

Interhospital transfer

Checklist for interhospital transfer

- *Airway with cervical spine control*—Use an endotracheal tube or Guedel airway if appropriate with a hard or soft collar. Give oxygen by a mask or T piece

- *Breathing*—Use an Ambu bag and appropriate connectors or portable ventilator (for example, oxylog)

- *Circulation*—Once intravenous infusion is established give plasma Hartmann's solution or Ringer's solution if hypotension develops

- *Dysfunction of central nervous system*—Send details of conscious level and central nervous system findings at base hospital with patient

- *Ensure* documents and radiographs are sent with patient

The events associated with interhospital transfer are a potent cause of avoidable mortality and morbidity after head injury. Problems are caused by:

- Delay in arranging transfer
- Inadequate resuscitation before transfer
- Inadequate preparation for the journey
- Inadequate care during the ambulance journey.

Patients with hypovolaemia who have not been fully resuscitated may become profoundly hypotensive during an ambulance journey. Patients in a coma should be accompanied by a doctor who has the experience and equipment necessary to carry out intubation and ventilation during the journey.

Outcome after severe head injury

Outcome at six months after head injury related to age, best coma score, and best pupil reaction at 24 hours after injury

	Dead or vegetative (%)	Moderate disability or good recovery (%)
Age:		
0-29	39	50
30-59	49	34
≥60	81	11
Coma score:		
3-5	84	11
6-7	56	29
8-10	28	58
11-15	16	72
Pupils:		
Both fixed	86	6
One or both reacting	16	72

The main determinants of outcome are coma scale score at admission, age, pupillary state, raised intracranial pressure, and the presence of hypoxia or ischaemia. About 40% of patients who are in a coma after initial resuscitation and beyond six hours after injury will die. Prognosis should not be estimated too soon because resuscitation and stabilisation may dramatically improve the patient's conscious level.

Late sequelae

Neurological recovery after severe injuries takes about two years but is most rapid within the first six months. Mental disabilities are far more important for the patient and his or her family than physical impairment. Personality changes, poor motivation, impaired memory and concentration, and lack of emotional restraint are the most common of these. They often cause difficulty with schooling, employment, and family relationships, and patients should be advised against returning to school or employment too soon after a head injury. Psychometric testing often discloses unsuspected difficulties and allows more directed rehabilitation to be formulated.

Head injuries

Moderate and severe deficits in patients with head injuries. Figures are percentages of patients

	Degree of overall disability	
	Moderate	Severe
Physical handicap		22
Cognitive impairment	8	78
Personality change	18	89

Common physical sequelae include ataxia, hemiparesis, speech disorders, cranial nerve palsies such as anosmia, unilateral blindness, diplopia, unilateral deafness, and tinnitus. Seizures occur in from 4% to 40% of patients, depending on the nature of the initial injury, focal injuries being more epileptogenic.

Symptoms after minor head injury

Proportion (%) of patients with certain neurological symptoms after trauma

	At discharge	At one year
Headache	36	18
Dizziness	17	14
Depression	8	18

The illustration of a skull fracture was reproduced from Rob and Smith's *Operative Surgery: Neurology* by kind permission of the publishers, Butterworth, and that of intracranial contents from *Neurology and Neurosurgery Illustrated* by kind permission of the publishers, Churchill Livingstone. Other illustrations were prepared by Mr Derek Virtue, medical illustration department, *BMJ*.

In a third of patients with minor head injury symptoms such as headache, dizziness, irritability, poor concentration, tinnitus, poor balance, fatigue, depression, and intolerance of alcohol will persist for more than six months. Many of these "postconcussional" symptoms are due to mild diffuse axonal injury, which occur in patients who have been unconscious for only a few minutes and who may have electrophysiological and neuropsychological abnormalities. The symptoms usually subside spontaneously; depression and anxiety may lead to their persistence but malingering is rare. When the symptoms begin only after an appreciable interval psychological factors are likely to be more important.

Specific treatment for postconcussional symptoms is lacking. In the early stages reassurance that severe brain damage has not occurred is important, but patients should not resume activity too rapidly: if the patient has difficulty in coping anxiety and depression may be provoked and lead to perpetuation of symptoms. Psycotherapeutic support is appropriate, but the value of more formal psychological rehabilitation is not proved. Analgesics are appropriate in the early stages, but the smaller their effect the greater the need for a psychological approach.

MAJOR MAXILLOFACIAL INJURIES

Iain Hutchison, Michael Lawlor, David Skinner

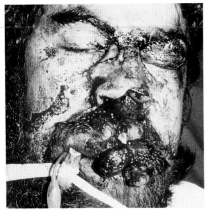

The multiply injured patient may have injuries of the face and neck that are life threatening or sufficiently serious to require specialist advice and management. In the initial assessment such patients may present with airway obstruction or hypovolaemic shock due to profuse and continuous bleeding from the facial skeleton or its surrounding soft tissues. The resuscitation team must be aware of these problems, know which specialists to call and when to call them, and be able to initiate manoeuvres to prevent the demise of the patient before the arrival of the specialist.

The first priority of the resuscitation team is to secure and maintain an airway, yet this action transgresses the site of maxillofacial trauma, which may be littered with broken teeth and dentures, bits of fractured bone, and macerated soft tissue.

Management of the airway

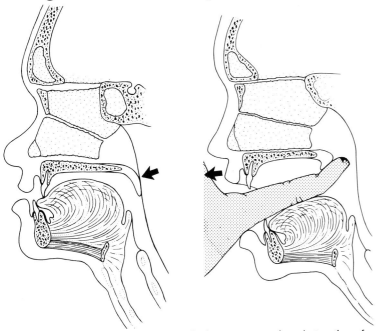

(Left) Fractured maxilla with posterior displacement, causing obstruction of the nasopharynx (arrowed). (Right) Fractured maxilla disimpacted and pulled forward to clear airway.

Six specific problems associated with maxillofacial trauma may affect the airway:

(1) A fractured maxilla may be displaced posteroinferiorally along the inclined plane of the base of the skull, blocking the nasal airway.

Management–Disimpact by pulling the maxilla forward with the index and middle fingers in the mouth behind and above the soft palate and with the thumb on the region of the incisors.

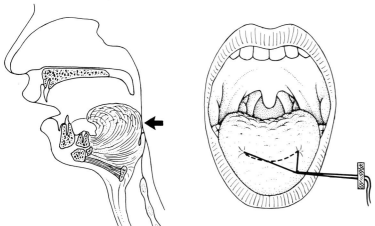

(Left) Fractured mandible with loss of anterior attachment of the tongue. The tongue drops back, blocking the airway (arrowed). (Right) Traction suture in the tongue taped to the face.

(2) The tongue may lose its anterior insertion in patients with a bilateral anterior mandibular or symphyseal fracture. It may then drop back in a supine patient, blocking the oropharynx.

Management—Insert a deep traction suture (0 gauge black silk) transversely through the dorsum of the tongue and tape the suture on to the side of the face; or, if no suture is available, pull the tongue forward by using a towel clip or pull the mandible forward manually.

Major maxillofacial injuries

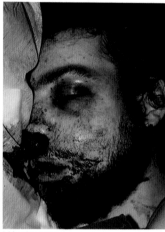

Life threatening haemorrhage from a closed bony injury of the maxilla.

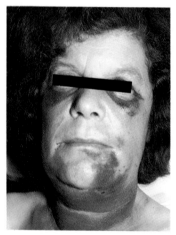

Haematoma and oedema of the neck and floor of the mouth caused by a fractured mandible.

(3) Teeth, dentures, bone fragments, vomitus, haematoma, and other foreign bodies may block the airway at any site from the oral cavity through the oropharynx, larynx, and trachea down to the bronchi, especially the right main bronchus.

Management—(a) Clear the oral cavity by using a gloved finger inserted laterally (just inside the cheek) to the back of the mouth, then hook the finger medially and forward to pull debris out of the mouth. (If the finger is pushed centrally foreign bodies may be pushed further down the airway.) (b) Repeat this manoeuvre from the opposite side of the mouth. (c) Use a large bore sucker (plastic yankauer) and good illumination to aspirate the oral cavity. (d) Use the laryngoscope and sucker (ignoring potential pain from mandibular fractures) to examine and clean the oropharynx and larynx.

(4) Haemorrhage may result from several causes:

(i) Distinct vessels in open wounds.

Management—Insert 5 cm ribbon gauze or gauze swabs as a firm compressed pack into the open wound to achieve pressure, request cross matching of blood, and arrange for definitive treatment.

(ii) The nose, as a result of damage to the anterior or posterior ethmoidal vessels or the terminal portion of the maxillary artery (see management of bleeding).

After dealing with these immediate problems consider orotracheal intubation.

(5) Soft tissue swelling and oedema. Trauma of the oral cavity causes swelling around the upper airway. This rarely presents an immediate problem, but the swelling may worsen insidiously over a few hours and cause later airway problems.

(6) Maxillofacial trauma may occasionally be associated with trauma to the larynx and trachea, which may cause obstruction of the airway by swelling or displacement of structures such as the epiglottis, arytenoid cartilages, and vocal cords.

Management—(a) Maintain a high index of suspicion if the mechanism of injury suggests trauma to the larynx and trachea: for example, in cases of blunt trauma of the neck caused by impact with a steering wheel. (b) Note any neck swelling, dyspnoea, voice alteration, and frothy haemorrhage. (c) Palpate the neck for surgical emphysema (crackling), tenderness, and, before swelling progresses, laryngeal or tracheal crepitus at the site of the fracture. (d) Arrange for lateral and anteroposterior radiographs of the soft tissues of the neck and mediastinum to be taken urgently to find out whether there is air in the soft tissue. (e) If suspicion is maintained perform bronchoscopy to determine the site of injury.

Management of bleeding

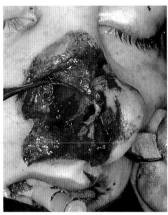

Apparently simple nasal soft tissue injury, which on exploration required extensive repair.

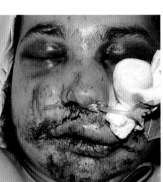

Major haemorrhage caused by closed maxillofacial trauma, treated by anterior and posterior nasal packing.

Procedure for anterior and posterior nasal packing

(1) Insert 12/14 G Foley catheters with 20 ml balloons into the nose

(2) Inflate balloons when the tip of the catheter is in the postnasal space

(3) Pull back the catheter until the balloon occludes against the choana at the back of the nose

(4) Tape the catheters under tension to the side of the face

(5) Insert bismuth iodoform paraffin paste 5 cm ribbon gauze packs into the nose in front of the balloon and Foley catheter

---

Secondary survey

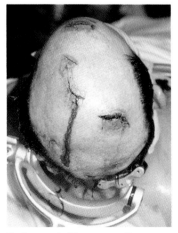

Underneath this apparently minor scalp injury was a fractured skull.

Soft tissues

Although the scalp, face, and neck have an excellent blood supply, extensive superficial lacerations in this region are not always accompanied by blood loss of such quantity that a transfusion is required. Conversely, small puncture wounds to the skin that scarcely seem to need suturing may cause life threatening haemorrhage if they involve a moderate size artery such as the facial artery or superficial temporal artery. The danger lies in overlooking the continuous trickle of fresh blood from the puncture wound.

Management—These wounds should be dealt with by senior specialist surgeons. Initial management comprises application of direct pressure to control haemorrhage. Definitive management comprises: (a) Assess wounds regularly for blood loss. (b) If haemorrhage continues explore the wounds and clip or ligate bleeding vessels. (c) Extend puncture wounds along natural skin crease lines to locate bleeding vessels. (d) If profuse bleeding occurs from a neck wound, consider whether there is enough time for arteriography, check arm pulses, extend the wound to expose the major vessels in the neck (usually along the anterior border of the sternomastoid), control the bleeding, and assess damage. Small vessels off the external carotid artery may be ligated. Large arteries (for example, the carotid and subclavian arteries) usually require repair. It is possible to ligate one internal jugular vein without untoward effect, and it may be possible to ligate one common carotid artery without causing a stroke.

Bone

Significant haemorrhage also occurs occasionally in patients with closed injuries to the bony structures of the middle third of the face—that is, the maxilla, nose, and ethmoids. This presents as a steady flow of blood from the nose and oral cavity and bleeding into the soft tissues of the face, producing profound cheek swelling with a shiny, tense skin.
Two problems exist:
(i) Failure to recognise the extent of blood loss and subsequent development of a coagulopathy.
(ii) An inability to define the source of the arterial bleeding as fractures of the middle third face are usually bilateral with disruption of the nasal septum. Therefore, haemorrhage from one side manifests equally at both nostrils.

Management—Exclude the possibility of bleeding from the base of skull by palpating the pharyngeal wall with your index finger through the mouth for tears and fractures. (b) Insert anterior and posterior nasal packs.

Once the airway has been secured and haemorrhage arrested the definitive management of soft tissue and bone trauma of the face and neck may be deferred until life threatening neurosurgical, thoracic, abdominal, and neurovascular limb injuries have been dealt with. It may be appropriate, however, to perform simultaneous procedures or even combined operations, particularly when cranial trauma is combined with facial trauma.

Examination

(1) Expose the affected area by cleaning all wounds and the face and scalp with Savlon (0·15% cetrimide). **Do not discard any loose bone or soft tissue fragments.**

(2) Examine the scalp for lacerations and bruises, not forgetting the back of the scalp if it is possible to move the patient—that is, if a cervical spinal injury has been excluded or the cervical spine is protected by a collar.

Major maxillofacial injuries

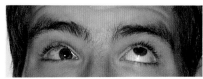

Limitation of upward gaze denoting an orbital floor fracture.

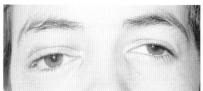

Proptosis and depression of right pupillary level due to fractured orbital roof and intraorbital haematoma.

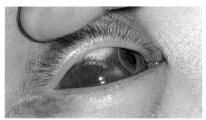

Subconjunctival ecchymosis.

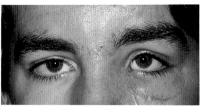

Left medial canthal damage with characteristic almond shaped palpebral fissure and increased intercanthal distance.

Indications of bleeding from the ears

Site	Indication
Anterior wall of the external auditory meatus	Fracture of the condylar neck of the mandible
Posterior wall or middle ear	Fracture of the base of the skull in the middle cranial fossa
Ecchymosis behind the ear (Battle's sign)	Probable middle cranial fossa fracture

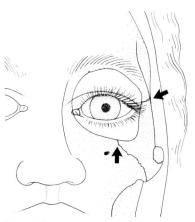

Palpate frontozygomatic and zygomaticomaxillary sutures for pain and separation.

(3) Examine the eyes for:
- Visual acuity—can the patient count fingers? Can he or she read print?
- Limitation of eye movements, diplopia, and unequal pupillary levels. If one or more of these is present suspect trauma of the orbital floor and wall with entrapment of periorbital tissues.
- Direct, consensual, and accommodation reflexes. Examination of these may help detect a rise in intracranial pressure, but be aware of false positive signs caused by trauma to the globe, resulting in post-traumatic mydriasis, and retrobulbar haemorrhage.
- Proptosis (or exophthalmos). This suggests haemorrhage within the orbital walls.
- Enophthalmos. This suggests fracture of an orbital wall (usually the floor or medial wall).
- Periorbital swelling. If this is present suspect a fracture of the zygoma or maxilla.
- Subconjunctival ecchymosis. If this is present suspect direct trauma to the globe or a fractured zygoma.

Examine the anterior chamber and fundus for evidence of direct trauma and raised intracranial pressure.

(4) Examine the nose for:
- Deformity, pain, mobility, and difficulty in breathing.
- Bleeding and leakage of cerebrospinal fluid. If present suspect anterior cranial fossa fracture at the cribiform plate. Do not pass a nasal endotracheal tube or nasogastric tube. Give prophylactic sulphonamides or chloramphenicol to prevent meningitis.

Measure the intercanthal distance. If it is >3·5 cm suspect nasoethmoidal fracture.

(5) Examine the ears for bleeding and leakage of cerebrospinal fluid.

(6) Examine the soft tissues for:
- Sensory (V nerve) (for example, of the upper or lower lip) and motor (VII nerve) deficit—this may have a peripheral or central cause. Consider this in relation to other injuries.
- Surgical emphysema around the eyes and on the face. This suggests continuity between sinuses and face due to facial fracture. To avoid emphysema instruct patients not to blow their nose. (Surgical emphysema in the face should be distinguished from that in the neck, which is caused by trauma to the larynx, trachea, or lungs)
- Venous engorgement of the face. If present suspect trauma of the major vessels in the thorax or neck.
- Pooling of tears and leakage from the eye. This may indicate damage to the lacrimal apparatus.
- Leakage of pink or clear fluid from a facial wound. If present suspect damage to the parotid duct.

(7) Examine the face for lengthening, bilateral swelling, "panda eyes," and dish face deformity.
If any of these are present suspect bilateral maxillary fracture.

(8) Palpate around the orbit for step defects, particularly at the frontozygomatic and zygomaticomaxillary sutures. Such defects indicate fracture to the zygoma or maxilla.

(9) Palpate the mandible externally from the condyle and along the lower border for tenderness, step defects, and crepitus.

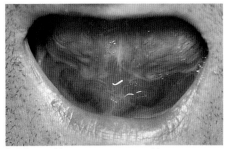

Sublingual haematoma caused by mandibular fracture.

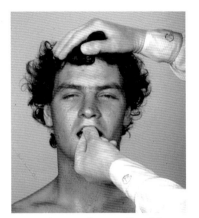

Pull on the anterior maxilla while supporting the frontal bone to show movement of the maxilla on the base of the skull, indicating maxillary fracture.

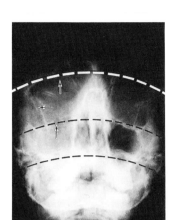

Anteroposterior occipitomental radiograph taken in the initial assessment period of a multiply injured patient. Examine along these standard arcs for evidence of fractures (arrowed).

(10) Examine intraorally for haematoma (especially under the tongue — this indicates mandibular fracture), lacerations, bleeding, loose teeth, broken teeth and dentures, mobile jaw segments, abnormal alignment of the jaw and step defects, and teeth meeting prematurely.

(11) Using both hands palpate the middle third of the face for mobility. Place the thumb and fingers of the right hand on either side of the premaxillary teeth (with the thumb in front and the index finger on the palatal side). Place the palmar surface of the left hand across the forehead. Pull the premaxillary segment forward gently and see whether nose or cheek bones move, indicating a maxillary fracture at the Le Fort I, II, or III level.

(12) Good quality maxillofacial radiographs help in the definitive planning of treatment. The radiologist will decide which views are appropriate.

Conclusion

The photographs of general facial trauma and limitation of eye movements were provided by Mr D R James, those of haemorrhage by Mr J Attenborough, that of proptosis by Mr R Haskell, and that of oedema by Mr R Juniper. The line drawings were prepared by the department of education and medical illustration services, St Bartholomew's Hospital, London.

Major maxillofacial injuries may occur in isolation or in combination with other injuries. They pose problems because they are intimidating and obstruct access to the airway. Rarely, they may be the cause of life threatening haemorrhage, which is often overlooked.

The definitive management of soft tissue and bone injuries of the face and neck can usually be deferred while life threatening thoracic, abdominal, and neurological injuries are dealt with. It may be appropriate, though, for the maxillofacial surgeon to help the anaesthetist and perform a fuller assessment, wound toilet, and preparatory procedures while the patient is anaesthetised. Combined procedures with specialists such as neurosurgeons may also be indicated.

TRAUMA OF THE SPINE AND SPINAL CORD

Andrew Swain, John Dove, Harry Baker

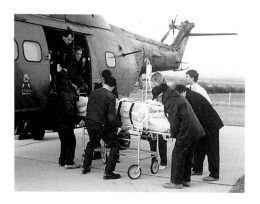

A patient with serious multiple injuries is rarely able to provide a coherent history. Injuries that carry a risk of death or severe disability must, therefore, be suspected from the outset so that correct early management can be instituted. Any patient with trauma who is not fully conscious should be assumed to have an injury of the cervical spine until proved otherwise. The thoracolumbar spine must also be managed carefully. The commonest reason for failing to detect an important spinal injury is failure to suspect one, particularly in patients with multiple trauma; but sometimes a serious injury is considered minor.

Incidence (percentage) of neurological injury in patients with fractures or dislocations of various parts of the spine

Part of spine	Incidence
Any	14
Cervical spine	40
Thoracic spine	10
Thoracolumbar junction	35
Lumbar spine	3

The spinal cord is most often damaged in the cervical region, but it is also particularly at risk near the thoracolumbar junction. The thoracic spine is splinted by ribs and sternum, but the spinal canal is narrower in this region relative to the width of the spinal cord so when vertebral displacement occurs it is more likely to damage the cord. Nowadays partial cord injuries are generally more common, and the potential for neurological improvement or deterioration is correspondingly greater.

Management at the scene of the accident

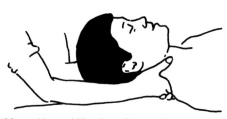

Manual immobilisation of the neck.

Spinal trauma may be suspected from a witness's description of an accident. It cannot, however, be excluded without a definitive examination, even in the fully conscious patient. The neck must be aligned in the neutral position without longitudinal compression or distraction. This will improve the airway and reduce spinal deformity, helping to relieve pressure on the spinal cord or arteries. If the patient is a motorcyclist the doctor should support the neck while an assistant carefully eases the helmet off. The neck is then splinted with a rigid collar of appropriate size to grip the chin. Collars alone are inadequate and they need to be supplemented by manual stabilisation or lateral support with, for example, sandbags and forehead tape. Be wary of swelling under the collar, which may develop from a haematoma or surgical emphysema.

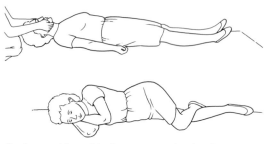

Supine position with airway protection (top); lateral recovery position (bottom).

In the unconscious patient the airway should be opened by chin or jaw lift and an oropharyngeal airway inserted. The supine position facilitates clinical examination, cardiopulmonary resuscitation (if required), respiratory movements, and control of the neck, but endotracheal intubation is required to prevent aspiration. Alternatively the patient can be turned into the lateral position with the trunk straight but inclined forwards by 20 degrees, allowing secretions to discharge freely from the mouth. The three quarters prone or coma position cannot be recommended as it entails rotation of the cervical spine and splints the diaphragm, causing hypoventilation.

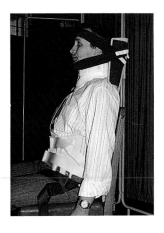

Semi-rigid collar and spine immobiliser.

Thoracolumbar injury must also be assumed and treated by carefully straightening the trunk and correcting rotation. The patient may be log rolled or lifted as necessary (ideally by five assistants), but it is vital that the whole spine is maintained in the neutral position.

The neck and back can be protected simultaneously in patients who are erect or supine by means of a spinal board or one of the more recently developed "spine immobilisers," which are lighter and easier to handle than a board. Doctors should familiarise themselves with the splints that are available locally.

Transfer to hospital

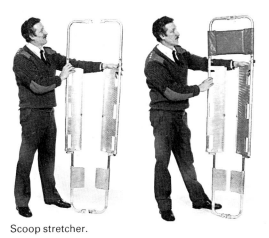

Scoop stretcher.

Once the airway is protected and oxygen has been administered and the patient positioned, one or more intravenous infusions are established. If conditions allow, the patient should be examined briefly before transportation. A "scoop" stretcher can be assembled underneath a patient who is lying free and used to transport him or her to the ambulance. Patients in immobilisers must be carried in and not by the splint. In the absence of life threatening injury the patient with spinal trauma should be transported carefully to hospital. Hard objects should be removed from anaesthetic parts of the body.

Arrival at hospital: primary survey

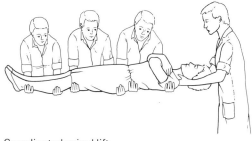

Coordinated spinal lift.

Safe transfer of the patient from the stretcher to a trauma trolley can be accomplished by four people, the person in charge grasping the base of the neck and supporting the head with his or her wrists. In this way there should be no seesaw movement of the neck if the actions of those lifting the patient become incoordinated. Once the patient is lifted the trauma trolley can be wheeled underneath. Resuscitation is then continued while the spine is protected.

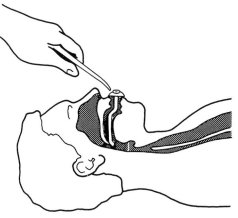

Suction: beware of vagal reflex stimulation.

Airway (with protection of the cervical spine)

Patients with multiple trauma are invariably kept supine during resuscitation unless regurgitation occurs and the airway is unprotected. In patients with cervical cord injury pharyngeal stimulation by vigorous suction manipulation of a Guedel airway or intubation may result in unopposed vagal discharge and cardiac arrest. This can be prevented by prior administration of atropine. Many seriously injured patients require intubation, and this is not contraindicated in patients with an unstable cervical injury. The procedure should, however, be performed whenever possible by an experienced anaesthetist and spinal movement minimised by an assistant controlling the head and limiting movement. Alternative methods of intubation that do not require the neck to be moved—for example, blind endotracheal intubation and use of a fibreoptic laryngoscope—should be employed only by those with the necessary experience. Ileus develops after spinal cord injury, and a nasogastric tube is required.

Treat

- Bradycardia—pulse rate <50 beats/min
- Hypotension—systolic blood pressure <80 mm Hg
- Inadequate urinary excretion

Do not rotate the patient's neck during central venous cannulation unless cervical injury has been excluded by radiography

Secondary survey

Causes of respiratory insufficiency

In tetraplegic patients

- Intercostal paralysis
- Partial phrenic nerve palsy—immediate
  —delayed
- Impaired ability to expectorate
- Ventilation-perfusion mismatch

In paraplegic patients

- Variable intercostal paralysis according to level of injury
- Associated chest injuries—rib fractures, pulmonary contusion, haemopneumothorax

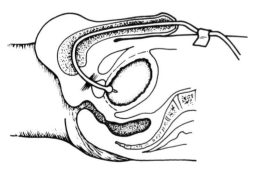

Method of catheterisation in patients with spinal cord injury.

Circulation

Patients with injury to the cervical cord or high thoracic cord may have reduced sympathetic outflow between the T1 and L2 segments with associated bradycardia and hypotension. Patients must be connected to a cardiac monitor on admission. Tetraplegic patients with bradycardia should be given atropine if their pulse rate drops below 50 beats/min. If their systolic blood pressure falls below 80 mm Hg inotropic support is necessary. Bradycardia with hypotension is not a classical feature of hypovolaemic shock, and in a traumatised patient it should increase suspicion of spinal cord injury. The extent of bradycardia and hypotension in neurogenic shock depends on the level and extent of neurological injury. Bradycardic shock is also seen in elderly patients and patients taking β blockers.

In recent years the importance of maintaining adequate tissue perfusion and oxygenation in patients with spinal cord trauma has been emphasised. Episodes of hypotension or hypoxia often lead to irreversible neurological deterioration. Patients with spinal trauma are likely to have hypovolaemia owing to other injuries. Circulatory volume must be restored, but aggressive fluid replacement is detrimental in patients with purely neurogenic hypotension as it precipitates pulmonary oedema (the commonest cause of early death in tetraplegic casualties of the Vietnam war). Therefore traumatised patients with bradycardia and hypotension should be subjected to a fluid challenge and the response observed and monitored by measuring central venous pressure. For this, cannulation of the subclavian vein is recommended as access to the internal jugular vein is difficult to obtain without rotating the neck.

Any injury to the spinal cord carries a high risk of early and late medical complications. Important early complications include respiratory failure due to intercostal paralysis or partial phrenic nerve palsy, impaired ability to expectorate, and ventilation-perfusion mismatch. The patient's respiratory state may also deteriorate shortly after admission as a result of ascending oedema in the traumatised cervical cord. Care must be taken in giving narcotic analgesics as these will further impair respiration. Cardiac arrest usually results from respiratory failure. Arterial blood gas tensions and vital capacity must be checked.

Abdominal trauma is not easily assessed in tetraplegic patients as the abdominal wall is anaesthetic, flaccid, and areflexic and ileus results from the neurological injury. A useful positive sign is pain at the tip of the shoulder that is aggravated by abdominal palpation. Peritoneal lavage is a particularly useful diagnostic aid in patients with cervical or thoracic cord injury.

Acute retention will develop in paraplegic and tetraplegic patients unless the sacral segments are spared. Measurement of urine output in patients with multiple trauma is important, and the bladder will usually require drainage, particularly if the patient has been drinking. In the absence of urethral trauma a narrow gauge Silastic catheter with a small (5 ml) balloon is passed under strictly aseptic conditions and taped to the anterior abdominal wall to prevent unnecessary movement of and injury to the urethra, which may lead to sepsis. Alternatively a suprapubic catheter can be inserted.

The conscious patient

Sensory loss or motor symptoms should never be disregarded, no matter how unimportant they seem. Diagnosis of spinal cord injury relies on symptoms and signs of pain in the spine with sensory loss and disturbances in motor function distal to a neurological level. The pain may radiate owing to nerve root irritation. A full neurological examination must be performed, including testing of cranial nerves, sensation to fine touch and pin prick, proprioception, power, tone, and reflexes.

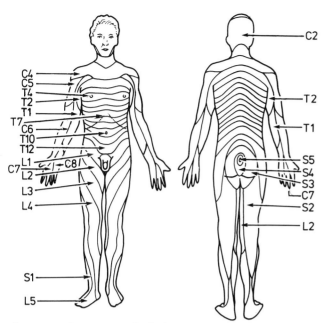

Sensory and motor neurological assessment.

Myotomes		Reflexes
Muscle group		*Nerve supply*
Diaphragm	C(3),4,(5)	
Shoulder abductors	C5	
Elbow flexors	C5,6	Biceps jerk C5,6
Supinators/pronators	C6	Supinator jerk C6
Wrist extensors	C6	
Wrist flexors	C7	
Elbow extensors	C7	Triceps jerk C7
Finger extensors	C7	
Finger flexors	C8	
Intrinsic hand muscles	T1	Abdominal reflex T8-12
Hip flexors	L1,2	
Hip adductors	L2,3	
Knee extensors	L3,4	Knee jerk L3,4
Ankle dorsiflexors	L4,5	
Toe extensors	L5	
Knee flexors	L4,5 S1	
Ankle plantar flexors	S1,2	Ankle jerk S1,2
Toe flexors	S1,2	
Anal sphincter	S2,3,4	Bulbocavernosus reflex S3,4
		Anal reflex S5
		Plantar reflex

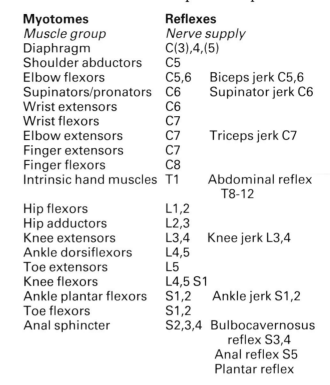

The central cord syndrome.

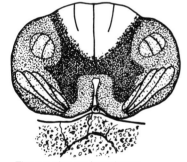

The anterior cord syndrome.

Great care must be taken in managing conscious patients as the neurological symptoms and signs may be dismissed if they do not fit a classical pattern. In patients with a partial cord lesion some neurological function is preserved distal to the level of injury (for example, the sacral segments may be spared): a vascular lesion may be responsible for this. Sometimes the zone of cord injury lies centrally, encroaching on the cervical segments of the long tracts and producing flaccid weakness in the arms (the central cord syndrome). Anterior contusion affects the spinothalamic and corticospinal tracts and is therefore associated with weakness and impaired pain and temperature sensation (the anterior cord syndrome). Posterior cord injury causes loss of sense of vibration and proprioception (the posterior cord syndrome). Trauma may be confined to one side of the cord, producing ipsilateral weakess and impaired contralateral pain and temperature sensation (Brown-Séquard "hemisection"). The central cord syndrome is more common in elderly patients in whom the spinal canal has been narrowed by cervical spondylosis. Patients with this syndrome may not have an associated fracture or dislocation, whereas those with anterior cord injury usually do. Brown-Séquard lesions are more common in patients with penetrating trauma and blunt rotational injury.

The unconscious patient

There are no truly pathognomic features of spinal cord injury, but important signs are flaccid paralysis, diaphragmatic breathing, priapism, hypotension with bradycardia, and upward movement of the umbilicus on tensing the abdomen—this is due to a T10 lesion (Beevor's sign). Examination of the *whole* length of the spine *must* be performed in all unconscious patients with multiple trauma. Failure to do so has resulted in diagnoses being missed, with serious consequences.

The patient is log rolled on to his or her side, keeping the spine in the neutral position. If performed correctly this is quite safe. Inspection may detect bruising, swelling, or a kyphos; palpation may allow tenderness, an increased interspinous gap, or malalignment of spinous processes (rotational deformity) to be detected. Suspicion of an injury to the upper cervical spine may be aroused by a retropharyngeal haematoma seen through the open mouth; the trachea may be deviated.

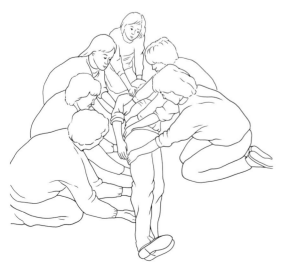

The log roll.

Trauma of the spine and spinal cord

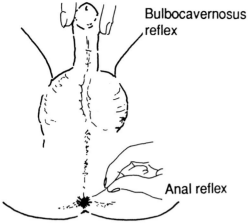

Bulbocavernosus reflex

Anal reflex

Sacral reflexes.

Neurological examination is mandatory in all unconscious patients, and baseline observations are extremely important in patients with spinal injury, not least for medicolegal reasons. Use of a Glasgow or similar coma chart will allow limb movements and strength to be charted. Some head injury charts do not include this facility. Neurological examination in unconscious patients is usually limited to completing the coma chart, funduscopy, and assessing tone and reflexes, but in patients with suspected cord injury the abdominal, anal, and bulbocavernosus reflexes should be recorded. The sensory response to pain can also be assessed in patients with depressed consciousness. Beware of flaccidity and areflexia in an arm as this may result from brachial plexus injury or spinal cord trauma, or both (particularly in motorcyclists).

Radiology

> ### Assessing spinal radiographs
>
> *Check*
> - Anterior vertebral border
> - Posterior vertebral border
> - Posterior facet margins
> - Anterior border of spinous processes
> - Posterior border of spinous processes
> - Integrity of vertebral bodies, laminae, pedicles, and arches
> - Prevertebral space
> - Interspinous gaps
> - For rotational deformity
> - All three basic views of cervical spine and two of thoracolumbar spine
> - Lateral view of sternum (for unstable thoracic injury)

Good quality radiographs are essential for accurate diagnosis of spinal injury, and these are best obtained in the radiology department if circumstances allow. When spinal injuries are suspected radiographic examination should be supervised by a doctor to ensure that there is no unnecessary movement of the patient. Collars, sandbags, and splints are not always radiolucent, and it may be necessary to remove them once preliminary films have been obtained. Riggins found that there was no radiological evidence of trauma in 17% of patients with spinal cord injury.[1] When in doubt seek a radiological opinion, especially with radiographs of children, which are difficult to assess.

Cervical spine

In a patient with multiple trauma radiographs of the cervical spine, chest, and pelvis are mandatory. If there is depression of consciousness skull radiographs or a computed tomographic scan of the head (if available) are required.

Most radiologically detectable abnormalities of the neck are shown in a standard lateral radiograph, which must display all seven cervical vertebrae if injuries are not to be missed. This can usually be achieved by applying traction to both arms, but pain in the neck or exacerbation of neurological symptoms must be avoided. If the lower cervical vertebrae are still not adequately shown a "swimmers view" and, if necessary, conventional or computed tomograms can be requested. These are helpful in excluding important lesions at the cervicothoracic junction.

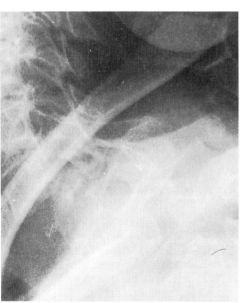

Swimmer's view showing dislocation of C6 on C7.

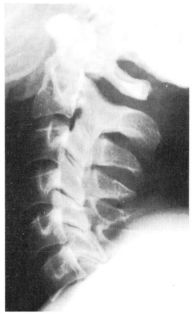
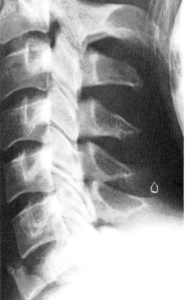

Compression fracture of C7, missed initially because of failure to show the entire cervical spine.

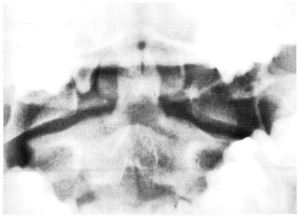

Open mouth odontoid view showing a Jefferson fracture of the atlas with outward displacement of the right lateral mass.

The lateral radiograph will normally show fractures, subluxations, and dislocations. Unilateral facet dislocation is associated with forward vertebral displacement of less than half the diameter of the vertebral body. This produces a change in the rotational orientation of the spine at the level of injury. Displacement of more than half the vertebral width normally indicates bilateral facet dislocation.

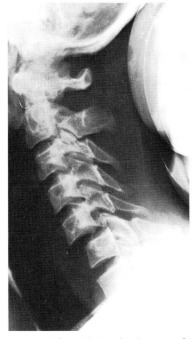

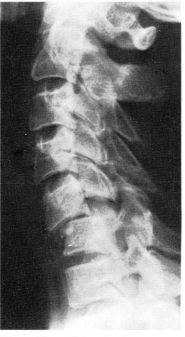

Unilateral facet dislocation between C5 and C6.

Bilateral facet dislocation between C5 and C6.

Many patients present with more subtle signs of an unstable injury. A chip fracture of the lower and anterior margin of the vertebra is commonly associated with a flexion injury, which may produce widening of the interspinous gap, loss of normal cervical lordosis, and minor subluxation. Always look for a prevertebral haematoma, which is indicated by an increased gap between the nasopharynx or trachea and cervical spine. The retropharyngeal space (C2) should not exceed 6 mm in adults or children, whereas the retrotracheal space (C6) should not exceed 22 mm in adults or 14 mm in children. (The retropharyngeal space widens in a crying child.)

The other standard radiographs of the cervical spine are the open mouth odontoid view and the anteroposterior projection. Abnormalities are more likely to be seen in the odontoid radiograph (for example, Jefferson fractures of the atlas as well as odontoid fractures), but the atlantoaxial joint must not be obscured by overlying teeth. In the anteroposterior radiograph look closely at the upper thoracic vertebrae and the first two ribs. Also take care to examine the alignment of spinous processes, which may be displaced laterally at sites of unilateral facet dislocation.

When standard radiographs are normal but cervical injury is suspected flexion and extension radiographs may be obtained later as long as neurological symptoms and signs are absent. Even these radiographs, however, may show no evidence of instability in children with cord injury or adults with cord compression resulting from spondylosis or acute disc prolapse. Rupture of the transverse ligament of the atlas is associated with an increased atlanto-odontoid gap, which should not normally exceed 2·5 mm in adults and 4 mm in children.

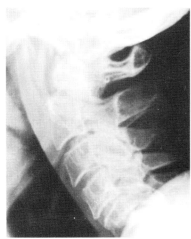

Odontoid fracture with posterior displacement of the anterior arch of the atlas.

Supine oblique radiographs of the cervical spine help to confirm the presence of facet dislocation if standard radiographs are difficult to interpret, particularly those of the cervicothoracic junction.

Trauma of the spine and spinal cord

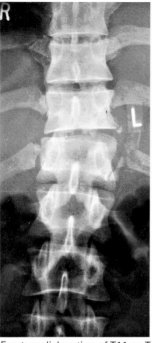 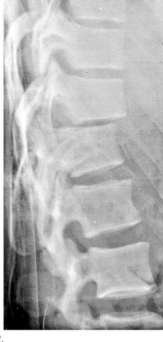

Fracture dislocation of T11 on T12.

Thoracolumbar spine

Anteroposterior and lateral radiographs are the standard radiographs of the thoracolumbar spine. Unlike a cervical haematoma a paravertebral haematoma in the thoracolumbar region is best seen on an anteroposterior radiograph, in which it may be responsible for mediastinal widening that resembles aortic dissection. In the lateral radiograph particular importance should be attached to subluxation, burst fractures, or potentially unstable fractures through the posterior vertebral complex (laminae and pedicles). The upper thoracic spine is usually difficult to assess in the lateral radiograph, and if symptoms or signs indicate, tomograms or computed tomograms should be considered.

Injuries of the thoracic spine can be rendered unstable by fractures of the ribs and sternum, which must be examined by radiography. An appreciable force is required to produce an unstable thoracic injury, which is usually evident in the standard radiographs.

Treatment

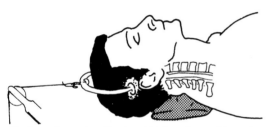

Skull traction using Gardner-Wells caliper with neck roll in position to maintain postural reduction.

Cervical injuries

At the district hospital orthopaedic surgeons should participate in the patient's management at an early stage. Unstable cervical injuries may be immobilised by a firm collar or skeletal traction. No technique is foolproof, and treatment should be supervised by a senior member of the medical staff. Skull traction helps to correct the alignment of the injured spine, reduce fractures and dislocations, decompress the cord and nerve roots, and provide stability.

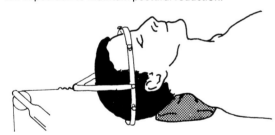

Halo applied with bale arm—an alternative approach to skull traction if early mobilisation into a halo brace is being considered.

Various skull calipers are available, but the Gardner-Wells caliper is easily applied, carries a low risk of complications, and has been used at the scene of accidents. In recent years halo traction has become more popular. Care must be taken not to overdistract injuries of the upper cervical spine, and for some of these traction is contraindicated.

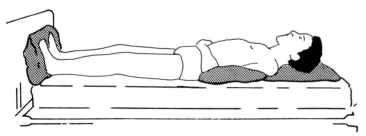

Conservative treatment for thoracolumbar injuries (postural reduction).

Thoracolumbar injuries

Thoracolumbar injuries may be treated by "postural reduction," which entails bed rest on a lumbar support to maintain the normal lordosis and help reduce the fracture or dislocation. Doctors commonly operate on patients with unstable injuries to enable them to be mobilised without much delay and to facilitate nursing care, though this approach is controversial.

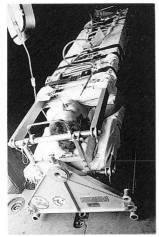

Patient immobilised in a Royal Air Force pattern turning frame for transfer to a spinal injury unit. Skull traction is maintained by means of the constant tension device.

Spinal injury associated with paraplegia or tetraplegia

Because of the medical complications associated with paraplegia or tetraplegia early referral and transfer to a spinal centre allows the patient to receive better overall care. Many spinal centres have intensive care units, and staff are experienced in dealing with complicated cases. Referral should be the responsibility of the orthopaedic or neurosurgical team. Routine administration of mannitol and antibiotics in these patients is controversial. However, the recent second national acute spinal cord injury study in the United States has shown that the degree of neurological injury may be reduced if very high doses of steroids are given during the first 24 hours after injury.[2] There is no conclusive evidence that surgery improves neurological outcome, but it is undertaken when there are signs of deteriorating neurological function and also to prevent deformity. The prognosis is always uncertain, and patients should therefore be treated actively.

Drug treatment in spinal cord injury

Give methylprednisolone at the earliest opportunity 30 mg/kg intravenously over 15 minutes and then 5·4 mg/kg/h for 23 hours

1 Riggins R. The risk of neurologic damage with fractures of the vertebrae. *J Trauma* 1977;**17**:126-33.
2 Bracken MB, Shepard MJ, Collins WF, *et al.* A randomized, controlled trial of methylprednisolone or naloxone in the treatment of acute spinal cord injury: results of the second national acute spinal cord injury study. *N Engl J Med* 1990;**322**:1405-11.

The illustrations of the lateral position, transfer to a trauma trolley, and log rolling were prepared by the department of education and medical illustration services, St Bartholomew's Hospital.

ABDOMINAL TRAUMA

Andrew Cope, William Stebbings

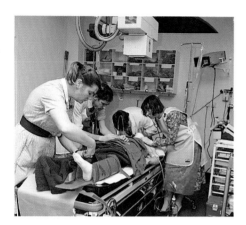

The aim of this article is to enable all those concerned with the management of patients with abdominal trauma to perform a thorough examination and assessment with the help of diagnostic tests and to institute safe and correct treatment.

Intra-abdominal injuries carry a high morbidity and mortality because they are often not detected or their severity is underestimated. This is particularly common in cases of blunt trauma, in which there may be few or no external signs. Always have a high index of suspicion of abdominal injury when the history suggests severe trauma. Traditionally, abdominal trauma is classified as either blunt or penetrating, but the initial assessment and, if required, resuscitation are essentially the same.

Blunt trauma

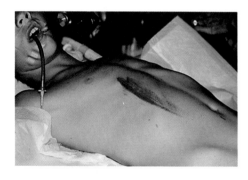

Road traffic accidents are one of the commonest causes of blunt injuries. Since wearing seat belts was made compulsory the number of fatal head injuries has declined, but a pattern of blunt abdominal trauma that is specific to seat belts has emerged. This often includes avulsion injuries of the mesentery of the small bowel. The symptoms and signs of blunt abdominal trauma can be subtle, and consequently diagnosis is difficult. A high degree of suspicion of underlying intra-abdominal injury must be adopted when dealing with blunt trauma. Blunt abdominal trauma is usually associated with trauma to other areas, especially the head, chest, and pelvis.

Penetrating trauma

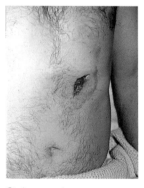

Stab wound.

Penetrating wounds are either due to low velocity projectiles such as knives or hand gun bullets or high velocity projectiles such as rifle bullets and shrapnel from bombs or blasts. With the increasing prevalence of civilian violence penetrating injuries, especially those due to stabbing, are encountered increasingly in accident and emergency departments. Visceral injury occurs in 80-90% of bullet wounds but only 30% of stab wounds. Penetrating wounds may seem easy to diagnose, but it is difficult to assess whether peritoneal penetration has occurred. About a third of abdominal stab wounds with serious visceral injury at operation have virtually no physical signs.

Assessment

> Remember the A, B, C of the primary survey

> To evaluate the abdomen Look, Feel, and Listen

Doctors must perform the primary survey—namely, airway management with protection of the cervical spine, breathing, and circulatory evaluation. The circulation may be compromised if there is concealed intra-abdominal bleeding. The usual diagnostic pathway of taking the history, physical examination, and special investigations cannot always be followed as resuscitation is the highest priority. The sequence of look, feel, and listen will help in the rapid initial evaluation of the abdomen.

Procedure

Information required in patients with abdominal trauma

From the patient or relatives and friends:

- Medical history
- Current medication
- History of allergies
- History of alcohol or drug misuse

From the police and ambulance crew:

- Speed of the vehicle
- Nature of the impact
- Evidence of deformation of the vehicle
- Evidence of steering wheel injury
- Whether a seat belt was worn
- Injuries to other victims

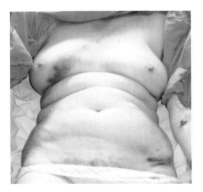

Seat belt injury.

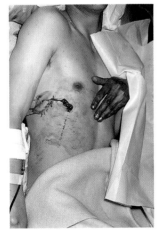

Anterior stab wound.

Signs of urethral injury

Blood at external meatus
High riding prostate
Bruised scrotum
Bruised perineum

Take a careful history

The patient may have limited recall of the injury owing to loss of consciousness, alcohol intoxication, or hysteria. Relatives and friends can provide information regarding medical conditions, current drugs, allergies, and alcohol or drug misuse.

In victims of road traffic accidents further information on the type of injury with regard to the speed of the vehicle, the nature of the impact, evidence of a steering wheel injury, whether seat belts were worn, and the condition of the other victims should be sought from the police and ambulance crews.

Useful information in patients with penetrating injuries includes their position when shot or stabbed and the length of the blade or the type of gun and the number and range of shots fired.

Perform a thorough examination

Look—You cannot perform an adequate assessment without exposing the patient fully; therefore you must remove all of the patient's clothes. Look systematically at the anterior structures, including the urethral meatus in men, the flanks, and the posterior structures—the back, buttocks, and perineum—for bruises, lacerations, entry and exit wounds, and impressions of seat belts or tyres. Any abnormality should be recorded.

Feel—Palpation, both superficial and deep, should include all abdominal structures. The abdomen starts at the level of the fifth rib, and therefore penetrating wounds of the lower chest can enter the abdominal cavity. The assessment of blunt trauma is difficult to interpret as muscle guarding results from intraperitoneal injury but can also be due to injury to the abdominal wall. Signs of peritoneal irritation after rupture of a hollow viscus can be slow to develop, and consequently the physical signs must be re-evaluated repeatedly. Abdominal rigidity usually indicates visceral injury; percussion and tenderness on coughing are also useful indicators of intraperitoneal injury. Instability of the pelvic ring can be confirmed by applying direct pressure in two planes to both anterior superior iliac spines. The superior pubic rami should be palpated in addition to the symphysis. Retroperitoneal injuries are difficult to diagnose but should be considered if there is a spinal deformity or paravertebral haematoma or if the mechanism of the injury suggests possible damage to retroperitoneal structures.

Listen—The presence or absence of bowel sounds and their quality if present should be recorded. The presence of bowel sounds does not exclude major peritoneal injury.

Rectal examination—Rectal examination is essential. Loss of integrity of the rectal wall and the presence of blood indicate trauma of the large bowel; a high lying prostate indicates urethral damage.

Vaginal examination—Disruption of the pubic rami or symphysis may cause vaginal injury, therefore, vaginal examination is mandatory, not only to confirm the integrity of the vaginal wall but also to detect obvious pelvic fractures, particularly of the inferior rami.

Examination of urethral meatus—In men the meatus should be examined for evidence of urethral injury. If there is blood at the meatus a urethral catheter should not be passed, and a urologist's opinion should be requested.

Once again the doctor must ensure that airway management with protection of the cervical spine, breathing, and circulation are adequate before proceeding to the special investigations.

Special investigations

Baseline blood tests

- Send a blood sample for cross matching, specifying the number of units required
- Measure haemoglobin concentration, white cell count, and packed cell volume
- Measure serum urea and electrolyte concentrations, serum amylase activity, and arterial blood gas tensions

Perform baseline tests

Determination of baseline haemoglobin concentration, white cell count, packed cell volume, and cross matching is essential in all victims of trauma. Blood for these tests may be obtained while an intravenous cannula of gauge 14 is being inserted. As a general rule it is safer to overestimate the amount of cross matched blood required. Biochemical measurements that should be made include urea and electrolyte concentrations, serum amylase activity, and blood gas tensions.

Pass a nasogastric tube

A nasogastric tube will not only empty the stomach contents but may also suggest upper gastrointestinal injury if blood is aspirated. The tube should be passed orally if there is a suggestion of a fracture of the cribriform plate.

Insert a urethral catheter

A urethral catheter is mandatory in all patients with severe trauma except those in whom urethral injury is suspected, when the suprapubic route should be used.

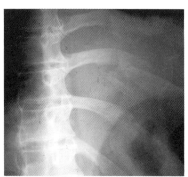

Fractures of the 10th and 11th ribs.

Perform radiography of the chest and abdomen

An erect chest radiograph is preferable to a supine abdominal film for excluding the possibility of free intraperitoneal air. Abdominal radiographs may show fractures of lower ribs, which may be the only sign of intra-abdominal damage, or fractures of the transverse processes, which may suggest ureteric injury. They can also confirm the presence of opaque foreign bodies (for example, bullets), confirm the position of the nasogastric tube, and show acute gastric dilatation.

In multisystem trauma radiography of the lateral cervical spine and pelvis is also performed.

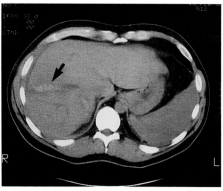

Computed tomogram showing liver laceration.

Additional imaging

Imaging techniques such as ultrasonography and computed tomography are not usually available for routine diagnosis in an accident and emergency department. Centres that have portable ultrasonic facilities should consider using them to assess possible subcapsular splenic haematomas or renal injuries. They should be used only after initial stabilisation and when there is no indication for immediate laparotomy. Computed tomography is valuable in diagnosing pancreatic and other retroperitoneal injuries.

Indications for laparotomy

Indications for laparotomy

- Unexplained shock
- Rigid silent abdomen
- Evisceration
- Radiological evidence of free intraperitoneal gas
- Radiological evidence of ruptured diaphragm
- All gunshot wounds
- Positive result on peritoneal lavage

If laparotomy is to be performed notify the most senior surgeon present and the anaesthetist immediately and alert the staff of the operating theatre.

Urgent laparotomy is required for profound hypovolaemia due to haemorrhage that persists despite adequate replacement of fluid volume when there is no overt cause (for example, haemothorax or a pelvic fracture).

Peritoneal lavage

Indications for peritoneal lavage

- Equivocal clinical abdominal examination
- Difficulty in assessing the patient because of alcohol, drugs, or head injury
- Persistent hypotension despite adequate fluid replacement
- Multiple injuries, particularly if they include injuries of the chest, pelvis, or spinal cord
- Stab wounds where the peritoneum is breached

If there is no indication for an urgent laparotomy peritoneal lavage may help you decide which patients subsequently require surgical assessment by laparotomy.

Contraindications

The only absolute contraindication for lavage is if there is already an indication for urgent laparotomy. Relative contraindications are pregnancy and previous lower abdominal surgery.

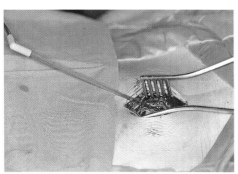

Peritoneal lavage.

Procedure

(1) Explain the procedure to the patient if he or she is conscious

(2) Ensure that a urethral or suprapubic catheter and a nasogastric tube are in place

(3) Prepare the patient's abdominal skin with antiseptic, and drape sterile towels over the abdomen

(4) Infiltrate the skin with a solution of 1% lignocaine and 1 in 200 000 adrenaline

(5) Make a vertical subumbilical incision in the midline 5 cm in length.

(6) Under direct vision divide the linea alba and identify the peritoneum

(7) Make an incision into the peritoneum and insert a peritoneal dialysis catheter (without an introducer) towards the pelvis

(8) Aspirate any free blood or enteric contents. If more than 5 ml of blood is aspirated an urgent laparotomy is indicated

(9) If no blood is aspirated infuse 1 litre of warm (37°C) physiological saline

(10) Allow the saline to equilibrate for three minutes and then place the bag and giving set on the floor with the tap open and drain as much of the original 1 litre as possible

(11) Send a 20 ml sample to the laboratory for measurement of white and red blood cell counts and for microscopic examination.

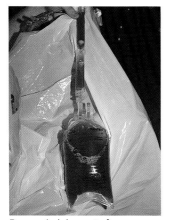

Bag and giving set after drainage of saline. The result was positive.

Interpretation of results

If >5 ml of blood or enteric contents is aspirated laparotomy is mandatory. If fluid from peritoneal lavage is obtained from either the urinary catheter or a chest drain an urgent laparotomy is essential.

Patients with a positive result must have a laparotomy. Patients with a negative result may be managed conservatively and should be frequently re-examined by the surgeon responsible for the case.

Positive result (one of the following)

Red blood cell count >100 000/mm³
White blood cell count >500/mm³
Presence of bile, bacteria, or faecal material

False positive results occur in about 2% of cases, particularly when the lavage is performed blind, and are caused either by trauma to vessels in the abdominal wall or by perforating a viscus with the trochar.

False negative results also occur in about 2% of cases. Most of these are thought to be attributable to injury to retroperitoneal structures and, occasionally, to diaphragmatic injuries.

Complications are rare but may include:

- Perforation of a viscus—for example, bladder or bowel
- Haemorrhage from mesenteric vessels
- Infection

Considerations for management

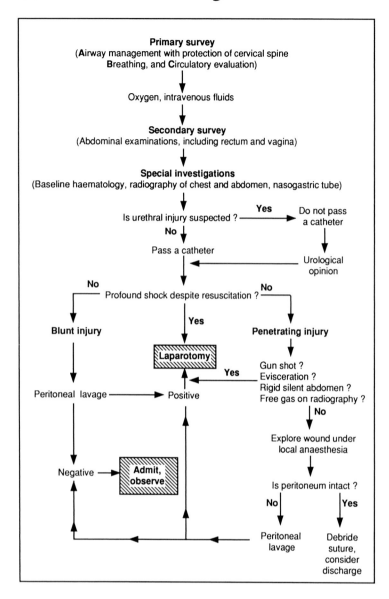

Primary survey
(**A**irway management with protection of cervical spine
Breathing, and **C**irculatory evaluation)

Oxygen, intravenous fluids

Secondary survey
(Abdominal examinations, including rectum and vagina)

Special investigations
(Baseline haematology, radiography of chest and abdomen, nasogastric tube)

Is urethral injury suspected ? — **Yes** → Do not pass a catheter

No ↓

Pass a catheter

Urological opinion

No — Profound shock despite resuscitation ? — **No**

Blunt injury   **Yes**   **Penetrating injury**

Laparotomy

Peritoneal lavage → Positive   **Yes** ←

Gun shot ?
Evisceration ?
Rigid silent abdomen ?
Free gas on radiography ?

No

Explore wound under local anaesthesia

Negative → **Admit, observe**

Is peritoneum intact ?

No   **Yes**

Peritoneal lavage   Debride suture, consider discharge

Penetrating trauma

All patients with gunshot wounds, regardless of the muzzle velocity of the gun, must have a laparotomy.

The tracks of stab wounds should be explored (not probed) to show the integrity of the peritoneum. If the peritoneum is not intact a laparotomy should be considered.

Lower chest wounds can be managed conservatively with careful monitoring, assuming that the results of lavage are negative.

Flank and back wounds are difficult to assess even with the aid of peritoneal lavage, ultrasonography, or computed tomography, and therefore laparotomy should be considered.

Evisceration of bowel warrants laparotomy.

Blunt trauma

In all cases of blunt trauma a high index of suspicion of intra-abdominal injury is essential. Blunt trauma is more difficult to assess clinically than penetrating trauma, and therefore diagnostic peritoneal lavage is helpful in evaluating the need for laparotomy.

If laparotomy is not required

Consider admission for all patients with suspected intra-abdominal injuries so that observation can continue. Such admissions will normally be to the general surgical ward, unless the patient's other injuries require intensive care.

Conclusion

The photograph of the trauma team was supplied by the department of education and medical illustration services, St Bartholomew's Hospital, and that depicting blunt trauma is reproduced from the advanced trauma life support™ (ATLS™) slide set by kind permission of the American College of Surgeons' committee on trauma.

Abdominal injuries should never be underestimated. In a recent retrospective study of 1000 deaths due to injury 43% of the deaths not related to the central nervous system were judged to have been potentially preventable. Among the commonest missed diagnoses were those of ruptured liver and ruptured spleen.[1] Thorough initial assessment and repeated re-evaluation with appropriate investigations are of prime importance for detecting these injuries.

1 Anderson ID, Woodford M, de Dombal T, Irving M. Retrospective study of 1000 deaths from injury in England and Wales. *Br Med J* 1988;**296**:1305-8.

TRAUMA OF THE URINARY TRACT

Timothy Terry, Anthony Deane

UPPER URINARY TRACT

> **Typical victims of urinary tract trauma**
>
> Young men while performing a sporting activity (55% of cases)
>
> People in road traffic accidents (25% of cases)
>
> Victims of domestic or industrial accidents (15% of cases)
>
> Victims of assault (5% of cases)

In the United Kingdom over 90% of renal injuries are a result of blunt abdominal trauma. Important associated injuries occur in about 40% of patients with blunt renal trauma. A high index of suspicion of a renal lesion is required in the patient with multiple injuries as the signs and symptoms of the renal trauma may be obscured by those of the concomitant injuries.

In children the kidney is the organ most commonly injured by blunt abdominal trauma. This may be explained by the relative lack of perinephric fat in children and the incidence (of up to 20%) of pre-existing renal abnormalities (primary pelviureteric junction obstruction is the commonest).

The mechanism of renal injury due to blunt abdominal trauma may be direct or indirect. With a direct injury the kidney is either crushed between the anterior end of the 12th rib and the lumbar spine—such as in sporting injuries—or between an external force applied to the abdomen anteriorly just below the rib cage and the paravertebral muscles—such as in run over accidents and injuries caused by seat belts and steering columns. Indirect injury occurs when a deceleration force is applied to the renal pedicle (as a result of falling from a height and landing on the buttocks). Such injuries can tear the major renal vessels or rupture the ureter at the pelviureteric junction.

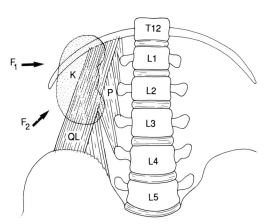

Mechanism of direct blunt renal trauma. An external force (F₁) may crush the kidney (K) between the 12th rib and the vertebral column, or a force (F₂) may crush the kidney against the paravertebral muscles (quadratus lumborum (QL) or psoas major in position P but deleted from diagram).

Penetrating renal trauma occurs in about 7% of patients with abdominal stab wounds. As with blunt renal trauma associated injuries are often present (in up to 80% of cases); these affect the liver, lungs, spleen, small bowel, stomach, pancreas, duodenum, and diaphragm in descending order of frequency. Renal stab wounds are potentially serious, with the possibilities of severed major renal vessels and lacerations to the collecting system or upper ureter. Gunshot wounds that involve the kidney may be caused by a low or high velocity missile. Low velocity missiles cause injury by directly penetrating the tissue whereas high velocity missiles produce direct tissue injury plus damage to adjacent tissue because of the shock wave effect see chapter on blast injuries.

Classification of renal trauma

> **Classification of renal injuries**
>
> *Minor (85%)*
> - Contusions
> - Superficial lacerations (capsule and pelvicaliceal system intact)
>
> *Major (10%)*
> - Deep lacerations (capsular tears or pelvicaliceal involvement, or both)
>
> *Critical (5%)*
> - Renal fragmentation
> - Pedicle injuries (renal artery thrombosis, vessel avulsion, and pelviureteric rupture)

Renal injuries can be classified as minor, major, or critical, based on the clinical and radiological assessments of the patient. Minor injuries (contusions and superficial lacerations) consist of parenchymal damage without capsular tears or involvement of the pelvicaliceal system. Major injuries (deep lacerations) consist of parenchymal damage with capsular tears or extension into the collecting system, or both. Critical injuries include kidney fragmentation and injuries to the pedicle (such as renal artery thrombosis, avulsion of renal vessels, and rupture of the pelviureteric junction).

Clinical presentation

Clinical signs of renal trauma

- Regional skin lesions (abrasions, bruising, and entry and exit wounds)
- Loin tenderness
- Loss of loin contour
- Loin mass
- Gross haematuria (up to 90% of cases)

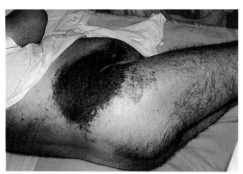

Severe abdominal and flank ecchymosis with potential urological injury (caused by a seat belt).

Radiological investigations

Findings on intravenous urography

Control film
- Fractures (of lower ribs and transverse processes of lumbar vertebrae)
- Loss of psoas shadow
- Loss of renal outline
- Loin mass (displacement of bowel or diaphragm

Postcontrast film series
- Distortion of caliceal pattern
- Contrast extravasation
- Non-visualisation of part or whole of caliceal system

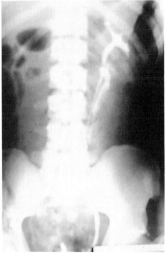

Excretory urogram with extravasation of dye.

Most patients (80-90%) with direct renal trauma give a history of a blow to the flank and complain of loin pain, which is followed after a variable period by gross haematuria. The haematuria may be subsequently accompanied by ureteric colic caused by the passage of blood clots. Clinical examination may show skin abrasions or bruising overlying the upper abdomen, loin, or lower thoracic area. Rigidity of the anterior abdominal wall and local loin tenderness over the affected kidney are invariably elicited. A flattening of loin contour together with a palpable loin mass indicate the presence of a perinephric haematoma with or without urinary extravasation of contrast dye. In such cases a paralytic ileus may be present. Varying degrees of hypovolaemic shock may be present, but this is usually secondary to associated injuries.

About 70% of potentially lethal injuries to the renal pedicle (indirect trauma) do not cause gross haematuria. Patients with such injuries are usually in severe shock, having been brought to hospital after a fall from a height. The same mechanism, in a milder form, usually produces intimal tearings of the renal vessels, which can lead to thrombosis.

The victim of a penetrating renal injury caused by a low velocity missile or stab wound will have an obvious entrance wound. The depth and direction of the wound track and the site of the exit wound, when present, suggest the likelihood of renal involvement.

The standard investigation in patients suspected of having a serious renal injury is intravenous urography. This includes all patients with gross haematuria and those with microscopic haematuria and a systolic blood pressure <90 mm Hg. Haemodynamically stable patients with microscopic haematuria have minor renal injuries and do not require urography.

The preliminary control film shows abnormalities in about 15% of patients with blunt renal trauma. These abnormalities include pneumothorax or haemothorax; concomitant fractures of ribs and the transverse processes of lumbar vertebrae; scoliosis with concavity towards the side of injury; loss of psoas shadow or renal outline due to perirenal haematoma; a soft tissue loin mass displacing bowel shadows or raising the ipsilateral hemidiaphragm; and free intraperitoneal gas. In 85% of patients with blunt renal trauma the postcontrast series of radiographs shows no abnormalities. The appearances in the remainder are those of distortion of caliceal pattern, extravasation of contrast dye into the perinephric tissues, or failure to visualise any part or the whole of the caliceal system. These findings suggest the presence of a major or critical renal injury, and the appearance in the intravenous urogram of a normal contralateral kidney is reassuring.

If patients with blunt trauma are clinically stable further information on the precise state of the damaged kidney (the presence of parenchymal disruption, intrarenal or subcapsular haematomas, and perirenal collections) may be gained by renal ultrasonography. This technique is particularly valuable for imaging injuries to the kidneys that are not visualised in the urogram and for following the natural course of perirenal collections. Computed tomography with enhancement with an intravenous radiocontrast agent, although a popular technique for investigating blunt abdominal trauma, is unlikely to give any additional information in patients with renal trauma over that provided by intravenous urography with nephrotomography and complemented with ultrasonography. Selective renal arteriography is indicated in patients with vascular pedicle injuries whose condition is stable and in patients with macroscopic haematuria persisting longer than one week. In the rare cases in which the mode of the accident and the findings on urography suggest the possibility of disruption of the pelviureteric junction a retrograde ureterogram is necessary.

Management

Management of renal trauma

- Treat hypovolaemic shock
- Stage renal injury radiologically
- Treat patients with stable minor and major renal injuries (up to 95% of cases) expectantly
- Operate on patients with critical and unstable major renal injuries

The principle underlying the management of patients with renal trauma is conservation of the maximum number of functioning nephrons with minimal morbidity and mortality. The immediate management of any individual patient is determined, however, more by the patient's general clinical state and the presence of important associated injuries than by the mode and type of renal injury. Less than 5% of all renal injuries are by themselves life threatening, and hypovolaemic shock in a patient with renal trauma is nearly always secondary to the presence of concomitant injuries. The initial general clinical assessment of the patient is thus all important in deciding a plan of supportive and definitive treatment.

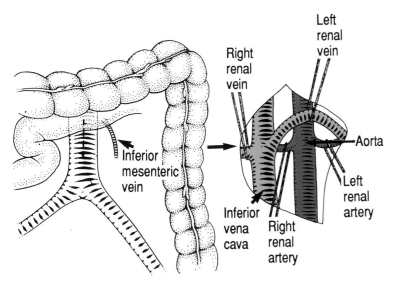

(Left) Retroperitoneal incision sited over the aorta medial to the inferior mesenteric vein to isolate the renal vessels before opening Gerota's fascia. (Right) The left renal vein crosses anterior to the aorta. With this vein retracted superiorly the left and right renal arteries may be located arising from the aorta.

In patients with blunt renal trauma urgent surgical exploration for critical injuries (renal fragmentation and pedicle injuries) is mandatory. A generous midline abdominal incision allows complete assessment of the abdomen for concomitant injuries while providing access to the entire length of both ureters, the kidneys, and the vascular pedicles. If conservative renal surgery is being contemplated the ipsilateral renal vessels must be isolated and controlled before Gerota's fascia is incised. Partial nephrectomy may be possible in some patients with fragmented kidneys, but usually total nephrectomy is necessary. Lacerations to the major renal vein may be debrided and sutured. If renal artery thrombosis has been diagnosed within 10 hours of injury thrombectomy, excision of the damaged arterial segment, and direct end to end reanastomosis may be considered. Disruption of the pelviureteric junction is treated by spatulation of the ends and reanastomosis over a ureteric stent.

Minor renal injuries (contusions and superficial lacerations) and major injuries (deep lacerations), which together comprise about 95% of cases of closed renal trauma, are initially managed expectantly. Strict bed rest, appropriate analgesia, and prophylactic antibiotics (cephradine or trimethoprim) are instituted together with frequent serial clinical observations of vital signs and assessment of any loin swelling. Once the vital signs are stable ambulation is allowed only after gross haematuria has cleared (serial aliquots of urine are kept for comparison) and the perirenal swelling, if present, has clinically resolved.

Expectant management of renal injuries

- Make serial clinical observations (pulse, blood pressure, temperature, urine aliquots, abdominal palpation)
- Institute strict bed rest
- Give appropriate analgesia
- Give prophylactic antibiotics
- Perform serial renal ultrasonography

Whether to perform early surgery in patients with major renal injuries is a controversial issue, but it is clearly indicated in those rare cases in which primary haemorrhage or secondary haemorrhage at 10-14 days, usually due to infection, endangers life. The late complications (after six weeks) of major renal injuries that may require surgery include hypertension, arteriovenous fistula, hydronephrosis, formation of pseudocysts or calculi, chronic pyelonephritis, and loss of renal function. Regular follow up is necessary in patients with major renal trauma during the first year after injury if these late complications, of which hypertension is the most common, are not to be missed.

Most penetrating renal stab wounds and all gunshot wounds involving the upper urinary tract require immediate surgical exploration to exclude or treat associated injuries, to assess and repair renal or ureteric damage, and to allow wound debridement.

Finally, an unsuspected penetrating or blunt renal injury may manifest itself at emergency laparotomy performed to control massive intra-abdominal bleeding in a patient with trauma. The clinically silent renal injury manifests itself as a retroperitoneal haematoma. In such cases on table intravenous urography is essential to establish the presence of a normal functioning contralateral kidney and to determine the type of injury to the damaged kidney. The retroperitoneal haematoma should be explored only if a critical injury is identified in the urogram or if the haematoma is large and is seen to expand during laparotomy. In either case the renal vessels must be controlled before opening Gerota's fascia, otherwise the possible use of conservative renal surgery may be jeopardised.

Late complications in renal trauma

- Hypertension
- Arteriovenous fistula
- Hydronephrosis
- Formation of pseudocysts or calculi
- Chronic pyelonephritis
- Loss of renal function

LOWER URINARY TRACT

Investigations in patients with lower urinary tract injuries

- Inspect the urinary meatus for blood
- Examine the abdomen for peritonism, perineal bruising, and a high riding prostate
- Perform intravenous urography to detect bladder perforation, displaced bladder, upper urinary tract injury

Perform cystography to exclude bladder perforation if patient has a catheter in place

Perform ascending urethrography (aqueous contrast) to exclude urethral injury (controversial)

Injuries of the lower urinary tract cause more confusion than those of the upper urinary tract as their management is controversial. The rule in patients with suspected urethral injuries and major pelvic fractures is not to pass a urethral catheter without first seeking advice from a urologist. Even though monitoring urinary output is very important in patients with major injuries, a catheter should not be passed without careful thought. Urinary extravasation is not dangerous in the short term.

Bladder injuries

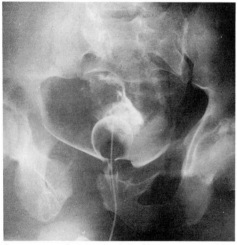

Cystogram of a bladder full of haematoma with extravasation of contrast due to a torn anterior bladder wall. The patient required 30 units of blood before bleeding was controlled by selective internal iliac embolisation.

Bladder injuries may be associated with a pelvic fracture—that is, they may be caused by penetration by a bony fragment or by a direct blow to the lower abdomen, especially when the bladder is full. The condition may be missed in patients intoxicated with alcohol or those with a head injury. Patients with a bladder injury may have lower abdominal peritonism and not be able to pass urine. A catheter may have been passed by the receiving clinicians and the urine may contain blood.

Investigation begins by obtaining a plain radiograph to exclude pelvic fractures. Disruption of the pelvic symphysis alerts the clinician to the possibility of urethral injury and delayed rupture of the bladder due to stretching of the anterior bladder wall. An intravenous urogram may show an extravasation from a bladder injury. If there is no pelvic fracture and no urethral haemorrhage a urethral catheter may be passed, and cystography with 10% dilute contrast agent will show any important bladder injury. If an intraperitoneal bladder rupture is suspected then cystography should be done before diagnostic peritoneal lavage because a laparotomy will be required to repair such a lesion, if it is present, making lavage unnecessary. In patients with serious pelvic fracture, especially if it affects the pubic symphysis, upward dislocation of the bladder on urography should be excluded first, although this would usually be accompanied by urethral haemorrhage.

Treatment—Patients with important intraperitoneal ruptures with peritonism are best treated by laparotomy and drainage by suprapubic catheter as well as by urethral catheter for about seven days. Broad range antibiotics should be given. Extraperitoneal injuries are managed by drainage by catheter without irrigation for about 10 days. A catheter of least 20FG is necessary, and cystography to confirm healing is advisable before withdrawal of the catheter.

Bulbar injuries

Management of patients with bulbar injuries

- Do not pass a urethral catheter
- If the patient passes urine give antibiotics and follow up
- If the patient has urinary retention insert a suprapubic catheter with a small calibre and give antibiotics. Perform urethrography after about five days and follow up

Bulbar injuries occur by direct trauma—for example by falling on to a bicycle crossbar. Occasionally thay can be caused by penetrating trauma. Patients with bulbar injuries have perineal bruising and blood at the urinary meatus. A urethral catheter must not be passed as it may aggravate the injury and introduce infection. The patient should be treated expectantly, and, if he or she passes urine, should be given antibiotics and followed up. Patients with urinary retention should be treated by inserting a suprapubic catheter with a small calibre percutaneously as heavy haematuria is not usually a problem. Antibiotics are given, and urethrography can be performed after about five days. The patient will need urological follow up to exclude formation of stricture.

Urethral injuries caused by pelvic fracture

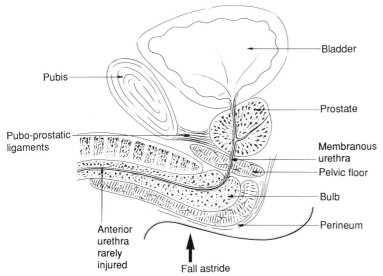

The puboprostatic ligaments carry the prostate with them in patients with pelvic fracture, tearing the urethra off the pelvic floor.

The membranous urethra below the prostate is damaged in about 10% of men with pelvic fractures. Serious injuries, though rare, are devastating as impotence and stricture are common sequels. Damage usually comprises a partial tear, but, occasionally, complete disruption and upward dislocation of the bladder and prostate occurs. The prostate is fixed to the pubic symphysis by the puboprostatic ligaments, and any severe disruption of the pubic symphysis is liable to tear the prostate off the membranous urethra, which is attached to the pelvic floor.

Signs of membranous urethral injury

- Pelvic fracture
- Perineal bruising
- Blood at the meatus
- Inability to pass urine
- High riding prostate

The signs of urethral injury caused by pelvic fracture are blood at the meatus, perineal bruising, and inability to pass urine. A urethral catheter must not be passed as it may aggravate the injury, even if it passes the tear: the urethra is often traumatised and devascularised and may be eroded by the catheter or disintegrate around it; the catheter will prevent the haematoma from draining and introduce infection with possible fistulation on its withdrawal; and worst of all, the catheter may pass out of the tear and drain blood and urine below the prostate. Balloon inflation may convert a partial disruption into a complete one.

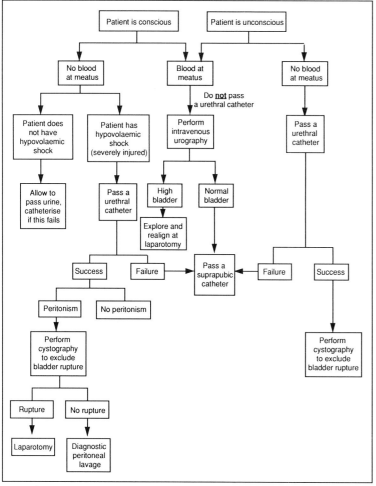

Urological management of men with serious pelvic fractures.

The safest way to treat urethral injuries caused by pelvic fracture is to pass a suprapubic catheter of adequate calibre either percutaneously or by cystotomy if the patient requires a laparotomy for other reasons or if the bladder is impalpable. Intravenous urography should be performed to exclude total disruption with a high riding bladder above the pubic symphysis—an indication for exploration and repositioning. Some authorities advise performing ascending urethrography to delineate the extent of the injury and plan its management, but this can be difficult in the emergency room. In general a urethral catheter can be passed in a patient with a pelvic fracture if there is no blood at the meatus or if the pubic symphysis is not severely disrupted on radiography. If any difficulties are encountered urological help should be summoned and an ascending urethrogram considered or suprapubic catheteris ation performed. If there is severe disruption of the pubic symphysis orthopaedic help should be requested as early fixation may assist in management and reduce morbidity. Later treatment of these injuries entails urethroscopy, but late strictures are very common.

In women the urethra is injured only rarely, and usually a catheter can easily be passed in those with pelvic fractures and, if necessary, cystography performed to exclude the possibility of bladder injuries.

External genitalia

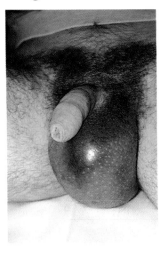

Scrotal haematoma.

Serious injuries to the penis and scrotum are unusual. The mobile scrotal skin can be used to cover penile defects and has good powers of recovery. Scrotal tears heal well without suturing. The erectile mechanism should always be repaired if torn with monofilament non-absorbable sutures.

The testicles can be damaged by direct trauma—usually a blow or a kick. If bleeding is confined to the scrotal skin no active treatment is required. Tense haematoceles should, however, always be explored as these usually indicate that the testis is torn and needs repair. Severe damage may require orchidectomy.

The illustration depicting ecchymosis and the excretory urogram were reproduced from the advanced trauma life support™ (ATLS™) slide set by kind permission of the American College of Surgeons' committee on trauma. The picture of scrotal haematoma was provided by Mr Andrew Cope, St Bartholomew's Hospital. The line drawings were prepared by the department of education and medical illustration services, St Bartholomew's Hospital.

MANAGEMENT OF LIMB INJURIES

Keith M Willett, Hugh Dorrell, Peter Kelly

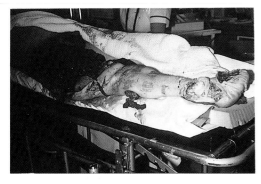

Up to 70% of multiply injured patients have injured limbs and fractures or dislocations of the appendicular skeleton. Severe limb injuries must not distract the resuscitation team from the priorities of establishing an airway, optimising ventilation, and restoring circulatory volume as limb injuries are rarely immediately life threatening, except those that cause exsanguination.

Careful thorough examination, however, is required after resuscitation to identify injuries, particularly those threatening the survival of limbs or fractures whose acute management will influence overall mortality or morbidity. Apparently minor injuries must likewise not be neglected as these may result in long term disability or disfigurement.

Prehospital care

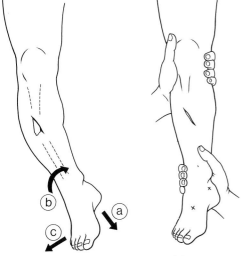

(1) Reduction of a major deformity; (a) perform gentle longitudinal traction) (b) restore the correct rotation; (c) restore the alignment.
(2) Control of the fracture; check pulses (×); maintain traction; apply a splint.

Doctors attending the scene of an accident should confine themselves to management of the airway and ventilation and immobilisation of the cervical spine and injured limbs. When moving a patient with a fractured limb the pain is reduced by supporting the limb on either side of the fracture and applying gentle traction along the axis of the limb. All unnecessary handling of the injured part without splinting should be avoided. The exceptions to this rule are when either severe deformity or ischaemia of the limb distal to the fracture threatens survival of the soft tissues; reduction is then indicated. This is achieved by gentle traction and restoration of the normal anatomical alignment. Perfusion of the distal limb must be checked after any manipulation. Prehospital care must avoid further soft tissue injury.

Splints are mandatory before the victim is evacuated, and anything rigid can be utilised—for example, pieces of wreckage, wooden sticks, etc. Strapping to the opposite leg is useful in solitary lower limb injuries, and "bulk" splints can be produced by bandaging blankets or pillows around the limb. Wounds should be covered with a clean dressing, preferably one that is sterile. External bleeding can be controlled by a compressive pad. Rapid transfer to hospital is then required.

Hospital care

Estimated blood loss caused by fractures

Site of fracture	Blood loss (litres)
Humerus	0·5-1·5
Tibia	0·5-1·5
Femur	1·0-2·5
Pelvis	1·0-4·0

For an open fracture the loss is two or three times greater.

Haemorrhage

Blood loss from limb wounds and occult bleeding from fractures contribute to the hypovolaemic shock in patients with multiple injuries. The accumulative haemorrhage from multiple fractures may result in exsanguination; patients with fractures of the femora and pelvis are at greatest risk. Patients with hypovolaemic shock should be resuscitated immediately with available crystalloid or colloid solutions while the dynamic response of the blood pressure and pulse is monitored. The total blood loss may be estimated (table), and blood for transfusion should be cross matched urgently. Blood loss from open fractures may be two or three times greater than that from closed fractures. Fractures, however, should not be assumed to be responsible for hypovolaemia, and occult bleeding into the visceral cavities should be excluded. Blood loss from wounds can be reduced by a compressive bandage or hand pressure over a sterile pad. A tourniquet is indicated only for unmanageable life threatening haemorrhage or after traumatic amputation.

Management of limb injuries

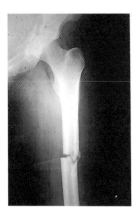

Acetabular fracture associated with a femoral shaft fracture.

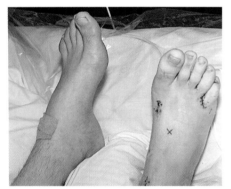

Ischaemic right foot.

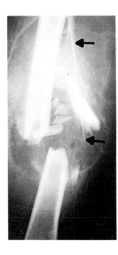

Femoral shaft fracture. Arteriogram showing occlusion of the superficial femoral artery at the level of the fracture.

Assessment

Evaluation of limb injuries is not started until the life threatening conditions have been treated. Careful examination is complemented by suspicions raised by knowledge of the mechanism of injury, information on which may be available only from attendants present at the scene of the accident. These witnesses should not be discharged until at least the mechanism, environment, time, and immediate care of the injury have been established. For victims of road traffic accidents it is important to determine whether they were a vehicle occupant, whether they were restrained by a seat belt, the direction of the impact, and the degree of damage to the vehicle. Ejection from a motor vehicle carries a high risk of serious injury.

Certain injury patterns are common. For instance, a direct blow to the knee in a seated occupant of a car may not produce only knee injury and femoral fracture but is commonly associated with hip dislocation or fractures of the acetabulum. A victim falling from a height and landing on his or her feet may sustain compression fractures of the calcaneum, ankle, tibial plateau, and one or more vertebrae at the thoracolumbar junction or in the lower cervical spine.

The patient must be completely undressed. The assessment should begin by comparing the injured limb with the uninjured limb. Observe the attitude of the limb: shortening and rotational abnormalities indicate proximal fractures or dislocations. Angular or rotational deformity may be visible or palpable. Clinical signs are often subtle, particularly in the unconscious patient, and careful inspection of the whole circumference and length of each limb for local swelling and bruising is necessary. Gently palpate along the axes of the bones and all of the surface bony prominences for tenderness, fracture crepitus (grating), and abnormal interfragmentary mobility. Carefully examine the adjacent joints so that coexisting injuries are not overlooked. A cooperative patient may indicate the active ranges of joint movement. Passive ranges of motion should be assessed cautiously in a limb that is suspected of being fractured; these should not be tested if an obvious fracture exists.

Vascular state

Of prime importance to limb survival is the competence of the vasculature distal to any injury. Local contusion, penetrating injuries, fractures, and, particularly, major joint dislocations may occlude or disrupt blood vessels. In the haemodynamically stable patient examination of the distal pulses is crucial in assessing the peripheral circulation. A diminished or absent pulse strongly suggests a vascular injury and must be explained and managed promptly. Skin colour will also indicate tissue perfusion, and pallor or a blue-grey colour should arouse suspicion. Similarly, a low skin temperature indicates inadequate perfusion. A sensitive indicator is the capillary return—the normal prompt pink flush of the nail bed seen after transient compression. This response will be slowed or blue if the circulation is inadequate.

Peripheral nerves are very sensitive to ischaemia, and sensation is lost early. Total insensibility in a hand or foot suggests ischaemia as, except in patients with injuries to the brachial plexus or spinal cord, it is unlikely that all nerve trunks will have been damaged primarily in one limb. An inadequate distal circulation is never due to spasm in a traumatised limb. If distal ischaemia is identified more proximal pulses should be checked and any major deformity at the fracture site corrected, the splint device checked for local compression, and an urgent surgical opinion sought. Dislocations of major joints require urgent reduction. Doppler ultrasonography may be useful in evaluating limb perfusion, but if a vascular injury is suspected arteriography provides the best definitive evaluation.

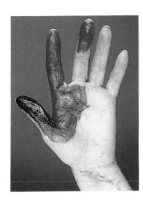

Areas of complete (black) and partial (red) sensory loss resulting from a wrist wound indicate damage to the median nerve, which was missed when the wound was sutured.

Neurological state

Evidence of nerve injury may be difficult to obtain in the unconscious or multiply injured patient. There is a higher incidence of neurological damage with dislocations than with fractures. Simple tests of sensitivity to touch, motor function, and sweating are sufficient to determine nerve integrity. When testing distal motor function the more proximal innervation of the muscle bellies must be appreciated. Division of a peripheral nerve must be assumed to have occurred if there is altered sensation in the distribution of that nerve and a wound overlying its course. Neurological function should be documented to allow later comparison.

Wound management

Management of wounds

(1) Obtain samples for culture

(2) Give preventive antibiotics intravenously

(3) Administer tetanus immunisation if necessary

(4) Remove particulate contaminants by physical wound cleaning and irrigation

(5) Excise all devitalised tissue

(6) Take a split skin graft early from skin flaps of doubtful viability

(7) Anticipate swelling, decompress compartments, and leave wounds open

(8) Obtain early rigid fracture stabilisation

Among patients with open fractures, 50% have multiple injuries. Correct management of wounds in the first few hours is decisive. The extent of the soft tissue damage will determine the outcome. A sterile dressing applied to an open wound at the site of the accident should not be disturbed. Definitive surgical toilet is required within six hours, and repeated examinations outside the operating theatre will considerably increase the risk of infection. Instant photography of the wound has been recommended to prevent this interference. As an adjunct to surgical toilet preventive antibiotics are indicated in patients with open fractures and contaminated wounds. A cephalosporin (for example, cefuroxime 750 mg three times a day) and gentamicin (80 mg three times a day) are appropriate and should be given intravenously for at least three days. Tetanus prophylaxis must not be forgotten and depends on the patient's previous immunisation state. An immunised patient with a contaminated wound that is prone to tetanus requires a booster dose of tetanus toxoid if more than five years have elapsed since his or her last dose. In addition, tetanus immunoglobulin is required if no immunity exists or the immunisation state is unknown.

Pelvic fractures

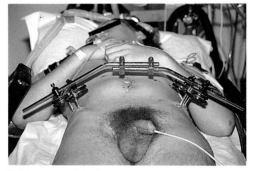

Pelvic external fixator.

Fractures of the pelvis are common in patients with multiple injuries and a radiograph is essential. The severity of these fractures is often underestimated: the fracture displacement visible in the radiograph may poorly reflect the disruption at the time of impact. A considerable force is necessary to disrupt the pelvic ring. The associated extensive soft tissue and visceral damage may result in life threatening haemorrhage. Damage to pelvic organs is common, particularly that involving the urinary tract. Urethral catheterisation should not be attempted if this is suspected because of the presence of blood at the urethral meatus, a perineal haematoma, or a high riding prostate on rectal examination. An urgent specialist opinion should be sought. Abdominal examination may be equivocal if there is a major pelvic fracture, and diagnostic peritoneal lavage may be useful. Urgent reduction and stabilisation with an external fixator will appreciably reduce blood loss in the patients with major pelvic disruptions.

Radiology

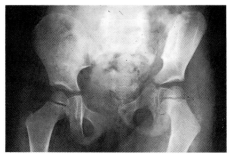

Vertical shear disruption of left hemipelvis.

Only when the multiply injured patient is resuscitated and stable and the three essential radiographs—of the chest, lateral cervical spine, and pelvis—have been performed should radiographs of limbs be considered. The standard two projections at right angles to one another are appropriate and must include the whole bone suspected of being fractured and the adjacent joints. Radiographs must be scrutinised for joint dislocations and subluxations that may be associated with fractures. Beware of requesting extensive radiographic studies if this requires the patient to be moved from the resuscitation area and its monitoring facilities.

Splintage

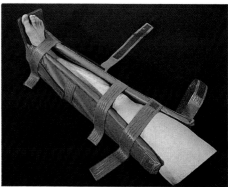

Leg splint.

The correct use of splintage will afford considerable pain relief, avert further soft tissue damage, and facilitate transport. To be effective the splint must immobilise the joint above and below the fracture and include the bone on either side of a dislocation. The arm is best supported by a simple sling and bandaged to the body. The forearm and wrist are immobilised on padded splints or pillows. The hand should be splinted in a functional position—that is, gripping a bandage roll. Femoral shaft fractures may be adequately controlled only by using fixed traction splints such as the Thomas splint or the modern equivalent. A traction force is applied to the leg or foot and is countered by a proximal pelvic bar. Low pressure (30 mm Hg) inflatable double walled polyvinyl jacket splints are now commonly used to immobilise tibial, ankle, and forearm fractures—they are easy to use and effective.

Compartment syndromes

Symptoms and signs of compartment syndrome

- Increasing pain—despite immobilisation of fractures
- Altered sensation in the dermatome of the nerve(s) passing through that compartment
- Palpable raised tension and tenderness of the muscle compartment
- Pain on passively stretching the muscles within the compartment

Beware:

- The pulses are often **present**
- Maintain a high index of suspicion in the unconscious or anaesthetised patient

Multiply injured patients with reduced tissue perfusion and oxygenation are at high risk of developing compartment syndromes. Increasing swelling in the unyielding fascial compartments, particularly in the forearm and lower leg, as a result of tissue contusion, bleeding, or ischaemia may result in autoinfarction of the compartment muscle. The clinical symptoms and signs are increasing pain, sensory deficit in the distribution of the peripheral nerves passing through that compartment, progressive swelling and tension, and pain on passive muscle stretching. The presence of peripheral pulses does not exclude an evolving compartment syndrome.

If signs of a compartment syndrome develop all potentially constricting dressings, casts, and splints should be released. If rapid recovery is not observed then prompt fasciotomy should be performed. A high index of suspicion must be maintained in the unconscious patient and continuous instrumented compartment pressure monitoring may be indicated. Compartment pressures of greater than 30 mm Hg are considered abnormal. It is a fallacy that compartment syndromes do not develop in patients with open fractures—an incidence of 15% has been reported.

Traumatic amputations

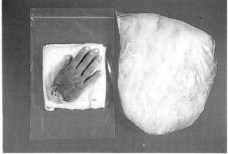

Management of an amputated hand.

Amputation is a catastrophic life threatening injury. Haemorrhage must be controlled as a priority. Replantation is possible in certain instances. In these cases the amputated part should be cleaned; wrapped in a sterile cloth that has been soaked in saline; and sealed in a sterile plastic bag, which is then immersed in a container of crushed ice and water. The limb must not be allowed to freeze. Rapid transfer to the definitive care centre is essential. Amputated parts that are unsuitable for replantation may be a source of bone, skin, vessel, and nerve grafts and should not be discarded.

Definitive management of fractures

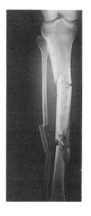 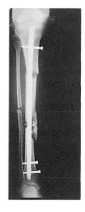

Internally fixed fractured tibia.

Closed fractures

The option of either surgical or conservative treatment of closed fractures available in patients with an isolated limb injury is inappropriate in the multiply injured patient. The incidence of, and the morbidity and mortality associated with, the adult respiratory distress syndrome, fat embolism, and late systemic sepsis are considerably reduced if the major long bone fractures are rigidly stabilised by internal or external fixation within 24 hours. This also results in easier nursing of the patient and a reduction in requirements for narcotic analgesia.

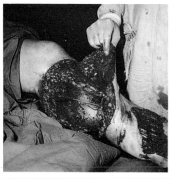

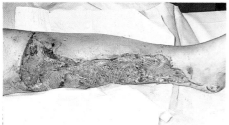

Soft tissue damage to the leg after a degloving injury (top); late flap necrosis was treated by excision and application of the split skin graft (meshed) obtained at the first operation (bottom).

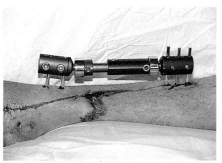

Externally fixed fracture.

Conclusions

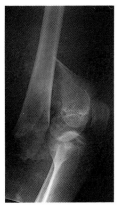 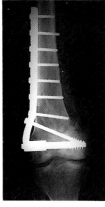

Unstable displaced supracondylar fracture of the femur (left); after internal fixation (right).

Open fractures

The soft tissue damage and the risk of infection are the two critical factors determining outcome in patients with serious open fractures of the limbs. The treatment employed in the first few hours can determine the difference between complete recovery and lifelong disability. In remembering that the infecting organisms are the contaminating organisms, samples for culture should be obtained at the outset. The priorities are to reduce the size of the infecting inoculum by physical cleaning and to ensure that all devitalised tissue is excised.

In a multiply injured patient with a reduced oxygen delivery and an anticipated rise in tissue pressure, wound hypoxia and an increased susceptibility to infection are inevitable. Closure of the wound is therefore rarely indicated.

Toilet of the wound is often performed inadequately. The surrounding skin should be shaved and particulate debris removed by scrubbing the wound with a brush. Meticulous exploration of the wound is necessary, and all recesses should be liberally irrigated by using a squirt and suck technique. Large volumes of warm saline or antiseptic solution are necessary (4-10 litres). Pressurised pulsed irrigation systems are now commercially available.

The wound is extended to facilitate examination as required. All non-viable muscle, fascia, and fat is carefully but radically excised. Fasciotomies may be performed once the wound has been thoroughly cleaned. Skin flaps of dubious viability are best dealt with by taking a split skin graft from the flap surface. This will serve to delineate the margin of viability, (the dead area will show no capillary bleeding). The harvested graft may be reapplied later if necrosis of the flap occurs. Small loose fragments of bone should be removed. Occasionally, large mechanically important fragments may be retained to help fracture fixation.

Most open fractures are unstable. Rigid stabilisation is now recognised to promote tissue healing. A variety of methods are employed; the application of an external skeletal fixator is currently the most popular; this facilitates wound access and nursing care. Closure of the skin defect within seven days with a split skin graft, myocutaneous flap, or microvascular free flap as appropriate will appreciably reduce the risk of infection and rate of non-union of these fractures.

The assessment and management of limb trauma should always be secondary to resuscitation and management of life threatening conditions. A knowledge of the mechanism of injury and careful examination are essential if all of the sustained injuries are to be identified. Assessment of the peripheral circulation is crucial to allow early detection and management of potentially limb threatening injuries. Appropriate reduction of fractures and dislocations combined with correct splintage will reduce pain and can prevent serious complications.

A high level of suspicion is necessary in the multiply injured patient to identify nerve injuries and detect evolving compartment syndromes. Frequent reassessment and recordings of the circulation and neurological function of an injured limb are essential. The seriousness of open fracture wounds should be appreciated and an aggressive approach to wound toilet adopted. Urgent operative fixation of the major fractures within the first 24 hours will contribute to a reduction in mortality and morbidity.

The illustrations of leg trauma were reproduced by kind permission of Mr A Cobb, Mr I Hudson, and Mr R Birch, and the radiograph of the pelvic fracture by Dr D Stoker. The pictures of the leg splint and amputated hand were taken by the department of medical photography, Royal National Orthopaedic Hospital, London. The line drawings were prepared by the education and medical illustration services department, St Bartholomew's Hospital.

RADIOLOGICAL ASSESSMENT

N M Perry, M D Lewars

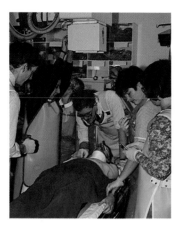

The mainstay of radiological investigation of trauma in the resuscitation room is the plain radiograph, which is available in all accident and emergency departments. Many immediate management decisions can be made with the aid of such radiographs, which show possible causes of cardiorespiratory compromise and detail any major bone or soft tissue injury. The development of pneumothorax, haemothorax, or early signs of aortic rupture may be clearly shown. Radiological investigation should not interfere with the mechanics of resuscitation or be allowed to delay appropriate surgery.

The experienced radiographer is an invaluable member of the emergency team. He or she can advise on the effects that positioning and resuscitation procedures may have on the images produced and give guidance as to possible delays caused by various radiographic techniques.

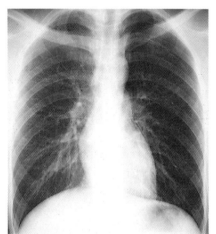

Left sided pneumothorax. The separated white line at the upper left heart border indicates pneumomediastinum.

Unnecessary exposure of the patient and, particularly, of members of staff to damaging ionising radiation must be avoided. Every radiograph should have a purpose. The quality of each image will depend on the time and effort taken to produce it. Full radiological evaluation may be deferred in patients with peripheral injuries that are not life threatening, particularly if there are other patients with trauma to be assessed.

Two important considerations in cases of major trauma are whether recognised focal injury has had hidden consequences and whether there is clinically occult damage that has been signalled early by radiography. For example, a rib or sternal fracture may be clinically quite apparent, but there may be an underlying haemopericardium; likewise a pneumothorax or pneumomediastinum may become apparent only on radiography.

Radiological survey

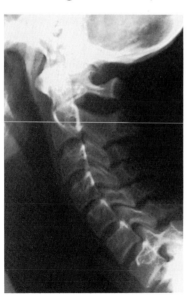

Normal lateral cervical spine radiograph of an adolescent showing smooth alignment and normal prevertebral soft tissue shadows.

Patients with major trauma should have immediate lateral cervical spine, chest, and pelvic radiographs taken, usually at the end of the primary survey or during the secondary survey. The images should be assessed as soon as they are processed and serve as a baseline for future comparison.

Every patient should be assumed to have an unstable cervical fracture until radiological and clinical proof of normality is available. The lateral cervical spine radiograph may be supplemented by anterior, oblique, and odontoid peg views if there is any specific history or clinical sign of cervical injury or if there is any abnormality in the lateral radiograph.

The patient is usually supine and immobilised by a variety of intravenous lines and airway tubes and by a stabilising cervical collar. These factors modify the quality of the radiographs. Some areas of the film may be overexposed (dark), necessitating the use of a bright light. Major trauma may affect different organ systems and parts of the body simultaneously. Once an abnormality has been identified and evaluated as far as possible attention should be turned to the possibility of an additional serious injury.

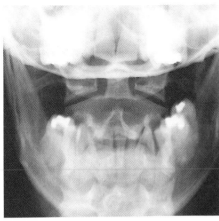

Supplementary "open mouth" odontoid peg radiograph showing symmetry of the lateral masses of C1 with regard to the peg and body of C2.

Many accident victims have had previous trauma or disease—for example, degenerative change in the cervical spine—which will be apparent in the radiograph. Age related osteopenia predisposes patients to fractures, especially vertebral wedge compression fractures. The age of fractures may be estimated from their density, cortical thickness, and trabecular continuity. In patients with major trauma it is safest to assume that all fractures are new. Familiarity with the variety of normal appearances can develop only with experience.

Two radiographs taken from different angles are required to assess any fractured bone: a single view rarely excludes a fracture. The bone contours should be inspected for irregular steps. Abnormal angulation, particularly in children, should be regarded as suspicious. With few exceptions (one being the knee) joint surfaces should be parallel and congruent.

Fractures are usually represented by lucent (dark) lines, which may or may not cross the entire bone. Occasionally, overlapping fragments may result in a linear density (white line) rather than lucency. Sometimes the only sign of fracture may be the alteration of the internal trabecular pattern.

Injured joints usually lead to effusions, even without fracture. Effusions may be visualised as soft tissue densities in relation to the joint capsule or by displacement of fat planes. Local haemorrhage from a skeletal fracture is also visualised as a soft tissue density with displacement or effacement of fat planes.

Soft tissue injuries may be more important than fractures, even when the two are associated. An atypical or asymmetrical soft tissue density may represent a haematoma or other fluid collection. The presence of gas in the soft tissues, visualised as dark streaks or bubbles in the tissue planes, is a sign of compound or penetrating injury involving the bowel, lungs, or neck structures.

Finally, if there is any doubt or mismatch of clinical and radiological appearances ask a radiologist for advice. Recent air, rail, and boating disasters have shown the advantage of experienced radiologists being present in the accident department: they are able to provide early authoritative interpretations of radiographs, direct the taking of further films, perform any necessary further investigation, and redistribute imaging services to accommodate the volume of work.

General principles of radiological assessment

- Plain films are most useful in the resuscitation room
- All patients with major trauma should have the following radiographs taken
  —Cervical spine (lateral)
  —Chest
  —Pelvis
- Imaging must not interfere with resuscitation
- Regard the cervical spine as unstable until proved normal
- Two views are needed to exclude bone injury
- Severe injury may be indicated only by soft tissue abnormality
- If in doubt seek radiological advice

Cervical spine

Features of the lateral cervical spine radiograph

- All seven vertebrae must be seen
- Check alignment of the spinolaminar, marginal, and interspinous lines
- Observe the anteroposterior depth of the spinal canal
- Look for localised or generalised prevertebral soft tissue swelling
- Check the predental joint space
- Look at the facet joints for superimposition or subluxation
- Check each individual vertebra for integrity of its body, lateral mass, laminae, and spinous processes
- Ensure disc spaces are regular
- Observe any displaced bone fragments

Any multiply injured patient must be considered to have a cervical injury. Manipulation or unguarded movement of the inadequately immobilised neck can cause cord damage, most commonly in patients with injuries below C3. A lateral radiograph shows 70%-90% of important cervical injuries. About 10% of patients with cord injuries have normal radiographs so clinical judgment may need to override negative radiographic findings.

Important cervical injury is associated with neurological damage in 40%-50% of cases; instability increases this risk by 10%-20%. Vital considerations are whether the radiological view supplied is adequate for assessment and whether there is evidence of either injury or instability.

Radiological assessment

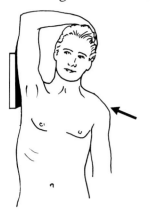

Position of patient for swimmer's view.

All seven cervical vertebrae must be visualised in the lateral radiograph. Injuries often occur at C6/7, with C1/2 next in frequency. The "swimmer's" view of the cervicothoracic junction is helpful when the lower cervical spine has not been fully visualised (see previous article in this series on trauma of the spine and spinal cord—II) but is difficult to interpret and is unsafe if cervicothoracic injury is strongly suspected as it requires manipulation of the patient. Anteroposterior oblique views with tube angulation of 30° will show the lower cervical spine and also the facet joints and foraminae. The patient need not be moved for these views.

Alignment of the lateral cervical spine radiograph
For each "line" work from T1 to the foramen magnum. Lines should be smooth with no angulation.

Spinous processes should be roughly equidistant and converge to a point behind the patient's neck. They should not diverge or "fan."

The spinolaminar line connects the white lines where laminae of each vertebra meet to form the spinous processes. C2 is frequently posterior to this line by up to 3 mm in normal subjects.

Anterior and posterior marginal lines connect the surfaces of adjacent vertical bodies and represent the sites of the longitudinal ligaments.

Prevertebral soft tissues—Above the level of the laryngeal inlet the prevertebral soft tissue should have a thickness of ≤7 mm. There should be no localised swelling. Below the larynx the tracheal air shadow should not be separated from the anterior marginal line by more than the equivalent of the anteroposterior diameter of a vertebral body: an upper limit of 22 mm is often quoted. Again there should be no localised swelling. Tracheal deviation in the anteroposterior view may be important providing there is no goitre present. Presphenoidal adenoidal enlargement in children and young adults may simulate a mass anterior to C1/2. Neck flexion and crying may also increase the depth of the prevertebral soft tissues substantially.

Vertebral canal—The anteroposterior diameter of the vertebral canal, measured between the spinolaminar and posterior marginal lines, is of prime importance at the site of cervical expansion of the cord—between C3 and C6. If it is <13 mm, particularly in the presence of bone injury, the cord is at risk or already damaged. Note any pre-existing degenerative cervical spine changes with osteophytes in elderly patients; cord damage can occur in these patients without noticeable narrowing. Likewise, spinal stenosis may be a longstanding feature due to posterior osteophytes.

Other observations
The space between the anterior cortex of the odontoid peg and the posterior cortex of the anterior arch of the atlas (the predental space) should be ≤3 mm in an adult (≤5 mm in a child). Greater distances imply atlantoaxial instability.
Disc spaces should be roughly equal in height unless there are associated degenerative changes. The height of any disc space should be even throughout. Angulation of >10° between apposed vertebral body end plates implies instability of traumatic origin.
Vertebral bodies should be inspected for evidence of fracture. The height of each vertebral body should be similar anteriorly and posteriorly. A difference in height of >2 mm between the front and back is important and may indicate a crush fracture. Fractures of the spinous processes are usually shown in the lateral view; fractures of the posterior arch, however, may be apparent only in oblique projections.

Important measurements in the cervical spine
- Predental space—≤3 mm (adult)
  ≤5 mm (child)
- Depth of spinal canal—>13 mm
- Depth of prevertebral soft tissue:
  Above larynx—≤7 mm
  Below larynx—≤22 mm (or depth of vertebral body)
- Overriding of vertebral bodies:
  Without fracture—25% indicates unifacetal dislocation;
  50% indicates bifacetal dislocation
  With fracture—>3·5 mm indicates instability

Signs of instability of the cervical spine
- Complete facet override
- Facetal joint widening
- Interspinous "fanning"
- Vertebral body compression >25%
- Angulation between vertebrae >10°
- Vertebral override >3·5 mm with fracture

Classification of cervical injury

Stable injuries
- Hyperflexion—compression fracture (if <25%)
- Spinous process fracture
- Unifacetal dislocation
- Pure C1 arch fracture
- Pillar fracture
- Lower cervical burst fracture

Unstable injuries
- Hyperflexion "teardrop" injury
- Hyperextension "teardrop" injury
- Traumatic spondylolisthesis of C2 (hangman's fracture)
- Bilateral facet dislocation
- C2 posterior arch fracture
- Hyperextension fracture dislocation
- Jefferson fracture of C1
- Basal peg fracture

A forward slip of one vertebral body on its neighbour may indicate dislocation. Shift of up to 25% of the anteroposterior diameter of the body is seen with subluxation and with unilateral facet dislocation. Displacement of >50% is a sign of probable bilateral facet joint dislocation. A forward slip of one vertebral body on its neighbour of >3·5 mm in the presence of a fracture indicates an unstable fracture dislocation.

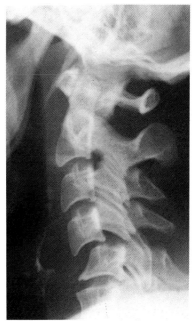

Forward slip of C4 on C5 of >50%. No fracture is present and the facets are overriding, indicating a bilateral facet dislocation.

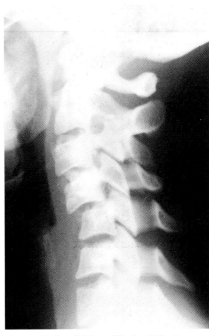

Forward slip of C4 on C5 of <25%. No fracture is visible. The disc space is slightly narrowed.

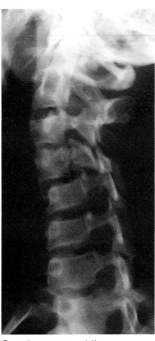

Supplementary oblique projection shows malalignment of the facet joints, indicating a unilateral facet dislocation.

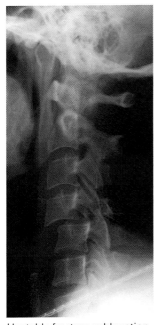

Unstable fracture subluxation. C4 has slipped forward on C5, the disc space is narrowed, and there is a fracture of the posterior elements and a fracture of the spinous process of C6.

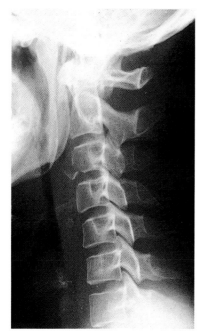

Hyperextension "teardrop" fracture of C3 showing avulsed anteroinferior fragment from the body of C3 and some localised prevertebral soft tissue swelling. This injury was unstable.

The two major mechanisms of cervical spine injury are hyperflexion and hyperextension. Hyperflexion is the commoner, causing 50%-80% of cervical spine injuries. There is a tendency for the posterior elements to be disrupted. Hyperextension injuries conversely tend to disrupt the anterior supports. "Teardrop" avulsion or compression fragments of the anterior aspect of a vertebral body may be the only residual features of major disruption and ensuing instability.

Compression fractures are generally stable. The Jefferson burst fracture of C1, however, is unstable, and the lateral radiograph may well show only soft tissue swelling. An open mouth view is essential to judge the integrity of C1 and the symmetry of its position either side of the odontoid peg (see chapter on trauma of the spine and spinal cord). C2 fractures may be associated. Neurological damage is rare as the canal is wide at this level. Conversely, neurological damage caused by stable lower cervical compression fractures is fairly common due to posterior displacement of fragments into a relatively narrow canal. A wedge fracture in an elderly patient with osteopenia should be differentiated if possible as it is unlikely to be important.

Radiological assessment

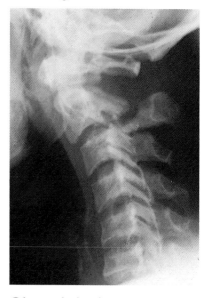

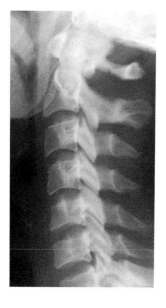

(Far left) "Hangman's" traumatic spondylolisthesis of C2. C2 is subluxed forward on C3 and the posterior elements are clearly separated. The posterior arch of C1 is also fractured. (Left) Pure C1 arch fracture. There is an undisplaced fracture line passing vertically through the posterior arch of C1. This injury was stable.

Fractures of the odontoid peg are commonest at its base. They are unstable, though neurological damage is uncommon. There is variable displacement, and soft tissue swelling is often seen only in the lateral radiograph. Ideally, a fractured peg should be excluded before intubation is attempted. An experienced anaesthetist may, however, be willing to proceed without radiological proof if the clinical situation dictates.

Chest injuries

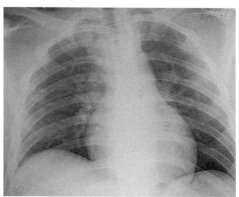

Anteroposterior supine chest radiograph showing poor inspiration and prominent upper lobe vasculature.

About 25% of deaths caused by major trauma are due to thoracic damage. The most useful radiograph in patients with thoracic trauma is the erect posteroanterior view. In the resuscitation room, however, the standard radiograph is often the supine anteroposterior view, which has the disadvantage of causing apparent enlargement of heart and mediastinal shadows, distending the upper lobe vessels, and making inspiration less efficient. In the supine position pleural air collects anteroinferiorly, outlining the diaphragm and heart, while pleural fluid layers posteriorly give ill defined opacification of the hemithorax.

Poor inspiration as well as rotation of the patient with relation to the radiographic beam may result in artefactually abnormal appearances. Ideally, five anterior ribs and 10 posterior ribs should be counted above the level of the hemidiaphragm. The medial ends of the clavicles should be equidistant from the vertebral spinous processes.

The basic rules for assessment of the chest radiograph are that the transverse diameter of the heart should not be greater than half the transverse diameter of the thorax and that two thirds of the heart should lie to the left of the midline. Vascular distribution should be symmetrical on each side, and each hemithorax should have equal translucency. The hilar shadows should be clearly defined, with the left hilum being about 1-2 cm higher than the right. Cardiac, mediastinal, and diaphragmatic contours should be clearly outlined.

Features shown in the initial chest radiograph

- Check for adequacy of inspiration, rotation of the patient, and artefacts of resuscitation

- Ensure that the density of each hemithorax is equal

- Localised opacities may be pulmonary, pleural, artefactual, or on the chest wall

- Look for rib fractures. How many ribs are fractured and how many fractures per rib?

- Check the mediastinum for contour, width, and presence of gas

- Check the aortic knuckle for contour and definition

- Look out for abnormal gas in the pleural, mediastinal, subcutaneous, and subphrenic spaces

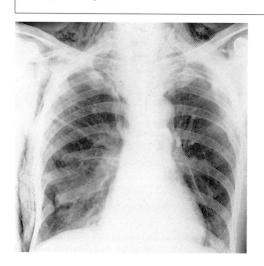

Chest wall injuries

Injuries of the chest wall frequently accompany pelvic trauma. The fifth to ninth ribs are most commonly injured. Lower rib fractures may be associated with splenic, hepatic, or renal damage, while fractures of the first two ribs imply that the patient has sustained a considerable force and is likely to have associated cranial, cervical, or intrathoracic injury. A fracture of the first rib with displaced fragments carries a 60% risk of underlying major vascular damage. The presence of surgical emphysema in the neck or mediastinum in addition highlights the severity of the injury.

Extreme surgical emphysema and pneumomediastinum caused by multiple rib fractures. There is outlining of the pectoral muscle fibres on the right side.

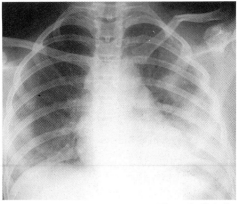

Left sided pulmonary contusion. There is ill defined opacification over the left mid-zone and base. Although the left clavicle is fractured, no obvious rib fracture is shown.

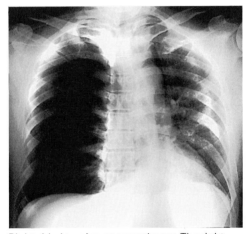

Right sided tension pneumothorax. The right hemithorax is very translucent with absent lung markings. There is flattening of the right dome of the diaphragm and considerable shift of the heart and mediastinum to the left.

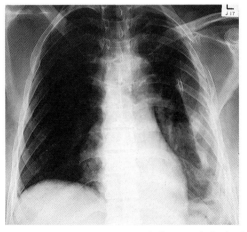

Flail chest caused by at least six fractured ribs both in the posterior axillary line as well as anteriorly.

Radiological signs of major thoracic trauma

- Mediastinal widening
- Mediastinal shift
- Mediastinal emphysema
- Multiple rib fractures
- Fractured first or second ribs
- Pleural fluid
- Loss of aortic definition

Flail chest occurs when multiple and adjacent rib fractures allow an area of the chest wall to move paradoxically with respiration. Sternal fractures are best shown in the lateral radiograph and may cause underlying pulmonary or cardiac injury. Posterior sternoclavicular joint dislocation can be identified by obvious asymmetry at the manubrium, and there is associated risk of brachiocephalic vein disruption. Complications caused by rib fractures include pneumothorax, haemothorax, and pulmonary contusion or laceration.

Diaphragmatic injury

Rupture of the diaphragm is commoner on the left side and can be caused by either blunt or penetrating trauma. Haemothorax, pulmonary collapse due to compression, rib fractures, and hepatic or splenic injuries may coexist. Ruptures due to blunt trauma are usually larger and more immediately apparent. The appearances are easily misinterpreted as a subpulmonic effusion, loculated haemopneumothorax, or just a high hemidiaphragm of unknown cause. A contrast examination may be necessary to show bowel loops within the thorax.

Major vascular and cardiac injuries

Major vascular and cardiac injuries may be found in association with sternal or first rib fractures and in patients with injuries caused by deceleration forces. Patients with aortic rupture may well survive to reach the resuscitation room. Vital features include mediastinal widening, loss of definition of the aortic knuckle, deviation to the right of the trachea, and thickening of the apical pleura on the left side (see previous article in this series on thoracic trauma).

Cardiac and pericardial trauma may cause haemopericardium with the risk of tamponade. The heart size will be increased, but classically described features of a globular appearance and notable clarity of cardiac outline due to reduced motion are unreliable.

Mediastinal injuries

Penetrating injuries may result in mediastinal or pericardial emphysema. This is apparent in the radiograph as a white line that parallels the mediastinal border, particularly on the left side. Free mediastinal air may extend to the neck, where streaky air lucencies are readily visible in the soft tissue planes. The tracheobronchial tree and oesophagus may be injured in patients with blunt, penetrating, or deceleration trauma. Oesophageal rupture typically causes mediastinal emphysema with an accompanying left sided pleural effusion. Bronchial fracture may cause segmental or lobar collapse but can also be very subtle radiologically.

Other findings

Sequelae of thoracic trauma include segmental, lobar, or pulmonary collapse. Features of opacification and alteration of hilar and fissure positions must be sought. Fluid aspiration causes patchy air space consolidation, typically in the upper lobes or apices of the lower lobe. Acute pulmonary oedema may appear solely as "bat's wing shadowing" extending from the hila resulting from fluid exudation into the alveolar spaces. Interstitial oedema is hallmarked by peribronchial thickening, the septal lines of interlobular fluid, and, indeed, pleural fluid. A pleural effusion may also indicate an abdominal injury such as splenic or hepatic laceration, and signs of subdiaphragmatic air from a visceral perforation should be sought in the chest radiograph.

Pelvic injuries

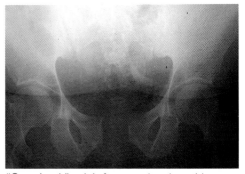

"Open book" pelvic fracture showing wide separation of the pubic symphysis and diastasis (widening) of the right sacroiliac joint.

The plain supine anteroposterior radiograph of the pelvis may be supplemented by radiographs of the inlet or outlet to show further detail of fractures or displacement. Judet views—acetabular views at 45°—may also be helpful.

General principles of symmetry and cortical and trabecular integrity apply to pelvic radiographs. Intrapelvic fat and soft tissue planes should be closely observed. Their displacement may be caused by large haematomas, which are common in patients with pelvic fractures owing to proximity of major vessels, venous plexuses, and considerable skeletal vascularity.

A single fracture in a bony ring with ligamentous support such as the pelvis should initiate the search for either a second fracture or a joint diastasis. Individual fractures may occur in the pubic rami, iliac wing, or sacrum.

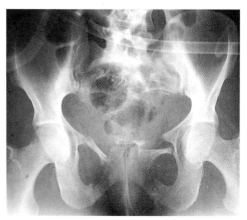

Bilateral pubic ramus fractures with separation (the straddle injury). Catheterisation for cystography has been performed. There is also an undisplaced left iliac wing fracture.

Fractures of the major pelvic ring are caused by different types of forces. Lateral compression may result in inward rotation of a hemipelvis with disruption of the sacroiliac joint. The pubic rami are usually fractured and sometimes the sacrum is also. Anteroposterior forces tend to drive the iliac wings apart and disrupt the symphysis (the open book fracture). Pubic ramus fractures may also be present. The straddle injury of bilateral pubic ramus fractures may be associated with urethral damage. Vertical shear forces tend to displace the hemipelvis upwards in relation to the sacrum, with high risk of vascular injury. Additional pelvic fractures will usually be present.

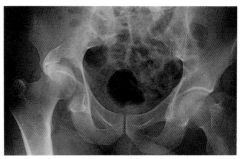

Acetabular fracture with posterior dislocation of the right femoral head. The acetabular fragment shows as a white line above the hip joint. The hip joint space is considerably widened medially and inferiorly.

The commonest type of acetabular fracture occurs in the posterior wall and is associated with posterior hip dislocation in a patient who has sustained a strong anterior force while in a sitting position. A lateral force may result in a central hip dislocation with associated acetabular fracture, but relocation either spontaneously or by manipulation may leave only subtle soft tissue changes. Anterior acetabular fractures are the least common.

A compound pelvic fracture may occur either with breaching of the skin or if bone fragments perforate the vagina or bowel. Such complication may raise the associated mortality to as high as 50%. Patients with pelvic fracture may require contrast examinations—for example, intravenous urography, urethrography, or cystography. Major pelvic trauma is associated with rupture of the bladder in 10-15% of cases.

Provided that the patient is stable, computed tomography provides excellent definition of the position of fragments, the acetabular anatomy, and any fluid collections. Arteriography may be used diagnostically or for therapeutic embolisation of bleeding vessels.

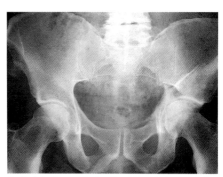

Left sided acetabular fracture with central dislocation of the femoral head. There is narrowing of the medial aspect of the hip joint space and medial displacement of the femoral head. Note the thick white line of overlapping bone fragments.

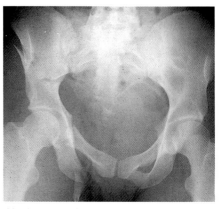

Vertical shear fracture involving both right sided pubic rami and iliac wing with a small amount of superior displacement. A sacral fracture is also visible.

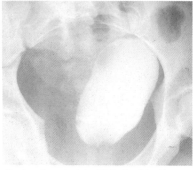

Contrast material within the bladder from an intravenous urogram shows bladder displacement by a large haematoma. The transverse sacral fracture can be clearly seen.

Skull injuries

Unnecessary importance is sometimes given to radiography of the skull. Criteria for its use have been proposed that essentially require that a neurological deficit of intracranial origin is present or that assessment of such a deficit is not possible. Some features to aid differentiation of fractures from other lucencies appearing in the skull radiograph are given in the table. Look carefully for the depressed fracture, which may be shown only by the white line of overlapping fragments.

Criteria for skull radiography

- Suspected penetration of the skull by a foreign body
- Cerebrospinal fluid or blood discharging from the nose or ear
- Loss of consciousness
- Altering consciousness during examination
- Focal neurological symptoms or signs
- Patient lives alone or is likely to be poorly supervised during the subsequent week
- Adequate clinical assessment is precluded by injury, intoxication, or a long standing clinical condition, such as stroke

Differentiation of lucencies in the skull

Feature	Artery	Vein	Suture	Fracture
Shape	Regular and roughly straight	Wandering	Tortuous but inner junction straight	Usually straight
Calibre	Even	Uneven	Even	Variable
Cortical margin	Present	Present	Present	Absent
Branching	Common, even	Common, irregular	Rare (for example, lambdoid suture)	May be stellate if depressed
Anatomical site	Fairly constant	Very variable	Constant	Anywhere

Other imaging techniques

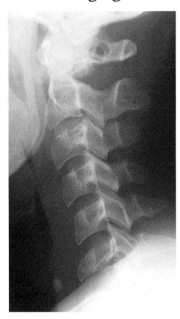

Apparent crush fracture of C6 with flattening of the vertebral body and loss of alignment of the anterior marginal line. There is considerable prevertebral soft tissue swelling.

Ultrasonography, computed tomography, angiography, and embolisation do not have a place in the resuscitation room, but they may alter the pattern of immediate management once the patient is clinically stable.

Ultrasonography may be used to assess damage to soft tissues, particularly in the abdomen. It can be used frequently in monitoring as it does not expose the patient to ionising radiation, though bowel gas and tenderness may preclude optimal imaging.

Computed tomography requires time for transfer and preparation of the patient, but this is repaid because minimum manipulation of the patient is necessary during investigation. The data obtained provide accurate assessment of the degree of internal damage as well as localising bone fragments and locating abnormal collections of air and fluid. The technique helps in determining the extent of spinal injury and compromise of the cord.

Angiography is used less often than previously because of the advantages of computed tomography but is better at showing vascular anatomy and may allow therapeutic embolisation to be performed.

It must be re-emphasised, however, that these are all further investigative radiological techniques that require the patient to be relatively stable. The plain radiograph remains the primary imaging technique in the resuscitation room.

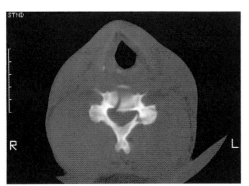

Axial computed tomogram through the C6 level shows not only the extent of the fracture through its body with some posterior fragment displacement but also a fracture through the arch (not apparent in the plain radiograph).

TRAUMA IN PREGNANCY

Pamela Nash, Peter Driscoll

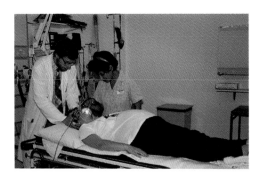

When a pregnant woman presents with major trauma two lives are at risk. Survival of the fetus depends on maternal survival. Treatment priorities remain the same as in patients who are not pregnant, although resuscitation and stabilisation should be modified to account for the anatomical and physiological changes of pregnancy. Early participation of an obstetrician is advocated.

If the patient is conscious she will be anxious about herself and her baby. It is important quickly to establish rapport with her. Allocation of an experienced nurse to this task will facilitate communication and allow other members of the trauma team to complete the primary and secondary surveys.

Anatomical changes

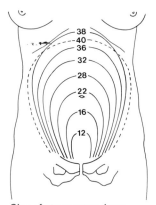

Size of uterus at various stages of pregnancy.

In the first trimester of pregnancy the uterus is a thick walled structure that is protected against injury by the pelvis. As the uterus enlarges to become an intra-abdominal organ it becomes progressively more vulnerable to injury. In the second trimester the fetus is cushioned by a large volume of amniotic fluid, but by the end of the third trimester the uterus is thin walled, offering little protection to the fetus.

Because, unlike the uterine wall, the placenta is devoid of elastic tissue shearing forces to the abdomen—for example, those caused by blunt trauma—may cause placental abruption.

Physiological changes

Physiological changes in pregnancy

Respiratory
- Tidal volume is increased by 40%
- Respiratory rate is unchanged
- Respiratory alkalosis

Cardiovascular
- Pulse rate is increased to 85-90 beats/minute
- Blood pressure falls by 5-15 mm Hg in second trimester
- Plasma volume is increased
- The aortocaval compression syndrome

Other changes
- Gastric emptying is delayed
- Risk of eclampsia

Airway
Ensure that the airway is protected at all times because during pregnancy there is relaxation of the gastro-oesophageal junction and delay in gastric emptying, both of which increase the risk of regurgitation and aspiration.

Breathing
The "physiological hyperventilation" of pregnancy results in respiratory alkalosis, with P_aCO_2 at term falling to 30 mm Hg. A P_aCO_2 of 40 mm Hg at this stage of pregnancy indicates maternal and fetal acidosis.

Circulation
During pregnancy blood volume increases by up to 50% and cardiac output by 1·0-1·5 litres. Compared with patients who are not pregnant, the pregnant woman has to lose a greater amount of blood before signs of hypovolaemia occur—that is, increased respiratory rate, falling blood pressure, and tachycardia (see chapter on hypovolaemic shock). Blood is shunted away from the uteroplacental circulation to maintain maternal vital signs.

In the supine position the uterus of a gravid woman causes pressure on the inferior vena cava; this impairs venous return, causing a fall in cardiac output of up to 40% and this may be sufficient to produce a fall in blood pressure (the aortocaval compression syndrome).

Primary survey

Primary survey

- **A**irway and cervical spine control
- **B**reathing
- **C**irculation (position patient to avoid supine hypotension)
- **D**ysfunction of the central nervous system
- **E**xposure

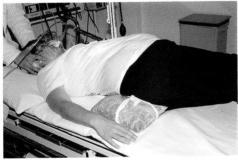

Patient with hip raised on a sandbag.

Control the airway, stabilise the neck, assess ventilation and give high flow oxygen through a mask-bag-reservoir system.

If an injury to the cervical spine is suspected immobilise the neck with a rigid cervical collar. Raise the right hip with a sandbag and displace the uterus to the left to reduce compression of the vena cava. Once spinal injury is excluded nurse the patient in the left lateral position to prevent supine hypotension.

Establish venous access with two large bore cannulas (14 gauge) in the antecubital fossae. Take blood for cross matching and determination of blood group, Kleihauer test result, full blood count, and urea and electrolyte concentrations. Vigorous fluid replacement should be started. Haemaccel has a product licence for use in pregnant patients and can be used before crossmatched blood is available.

If pneumatic anti-shock suits are used only the leg compartments should be inflated.

A rapid neurological assessment should be performed and all articles of clothing removed.

Secondary survey

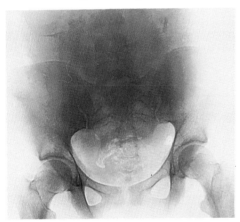

Radiograph taken after a fall excludes pelvic fracture.

Assessment of the fetus

- Note date of last menstrual period
- Measure fundal height
- Examine for uterine contractions or tenderness
- Examine for fetal movement
- Monitor fetal heart rate
- Perform vaginal examination for amniotic fluid or blood

Signs of fetal distress

- Bradycardia (<110 breaths/minute)
- Signs on cardiotocography:
  Inadequate accelerations in fetal heart rate in response to uterine contraction
  Late decelerations in fetal heart rate in response to uterine contraction

Assessment of the mother

Perform a head to toe examination of the mother during the secondary survey. Urgent radiography should not be withheld as the priority is keeping the mother alive. The radiation dose to the uterus can be reduced by minimising repeat of abdominal or pelvic radiography and use of lead abdominal shields when taking other radiographs.

Injuries should be treated in the same way as those in patients who are not pregnant. Peritoneal lavage can be performed if indicated by using a supraumbilical minilaparotomy approach after placement of a urinary catheter and nasogastric tube. If abdominal surgery is required this should not be delayed because of pregnancy.

The presence of a pelvic fracture should alert the clinician to the possibility of damage to the dilated pelvic veins and subsequent massive retroperitoneal haemorrhage.

Assessment of the fetus

Assessment of the fetus forms part of the secondary survey of the mother and should be performed in conjunction with an obstetrician because beyond 26-28 weeks' gestation the fetus is potentially viable if urgent delivery is required.

The normal fetal heart rate is 120-160 beats/minute. Fetal bradycardia and loss of beat to beat variation are signs of fetal distress. Doppler ultrasonography can be used to assess fetal heart rate from 12-14 weeks' gestation. Later in pregnancy the fetus can be monitored by cardiotocography; this compares fetal heart rate with uterine contractions. Signs of fetal distress include inadequate acceleration in fetal heart rate in response to uterine contractions and late decelerations in response to contractions.

Fetal gestation and viability can be confirmed by pelvic ultrasonography, the fetal heart beat being visible from seven weeks' gestation. Ultrasonography is also useful later in pregnancy to assess placental position, volume of liquor, and the presence of intra-amniotic haemorrhage.

The Kleihauer test is used to assess the presence and degree of fetomaternal haemorrhage after trauma. This can be used to predict fetal anaemia in utero. If fetomaternal haemorrhage occurs in a Rhesus negative mother prophylactic anti-D should be given to protect against Rhesus sensitisation.

Blunt trauma

Signs of placental abruption

- Vaginal bleeding
- Uterine irritability
- Abdominal tenderness
- Increasing fundal height
- Maternal hypovolaemic shock
- Fetal distress

Placental abruption is a common cause of fetal death after blunt trauma, second only to maternal hypovolaemic shock. Clinical signs are usually obvious, but fetal distress may be the only evidence. Because placental abruption may occur up to 48 hours after the injury fetal monitoring is advocated during this period to detect fetal distress in patients with appreciable trauma (especially abdominal trauma), vaginal bleeding, or seat belt injury. Major placental separation with or without amniotic fluid embolism can lead to disseminated intravascular coagulation.

In the late stages of pregnancy the uterus is susceptible to traumatic rupture. This has a wide range of presentations, from massive haemorrhage and shock to minimal symptoms and signs. The finding of a separately palpable uterus and fetus is pathognomonic.

Penetrating trauma

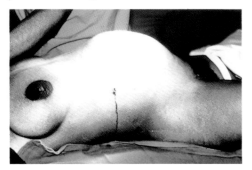

Penetrating abdominal trauma.

As pregnancy progresses the uterus becomes increasingly vulnerable to penetrating trauma, with the uterus acting as a shield for the other intra-abdominal organs. After gunshot and stab wounds to the abdomen fetal injury and death are common, but maternal survival is good because the uterus is a non-vital organ.

Burns

Immediate delivery is indicated when maternal burns exceed 50% of body surface area in the second or third trimester

Burns that affect more than 50% of the body surface area that occur in the second or third trimesters of pregnancy are associated with high maternal mortality. These patients should be delivered immediately as maternal death is otherwise certain and fetal prognosis not improved by waiting.

Conclusion

Indications for surgical or obstetric intervention

- Need for treatment of maternal injuries
- Penetrating abdominal trauma
- Uterine rupture
- Placental abruption
- Fetal distress at >26 weeks' gestation
- Burns affecting >50% of body surface area in second or third trimester
- Need for caesarean section after maternal death

The priorities in the management of the pregnant woman with trauma are the same as for patients who are not pregnant. The aims are to resuscitate and stabilise the mother and then assess the fetus, with early help from an obstetrician.

The photograph depicting penetrating abdominal trauma is reproduced from the advanced trauma life support™ (ATLS™) set by kind permission of the American College of Surgeons' committee on trauma. The line drawing was prepared by the department of education and medical illustration services, St Bartholomew's Hospital, London.

PAEDIATRIC TRAUMA

A R Lloyd-Thomas, I Anderson

Causes of childhood trauma

Age 0-1 years—Choking/suffocation, burns, drowning, falls

Age 1-4 years—Road traffic accidents (as occupant of vehicle), burns, drowning, falls

Age 5-14 years—Road traffic accidents (as occupant or pedestrian), bicycle injuries, burns, drowning

---

Trauma is the most common cause of death in childhood, with the aetiology of the injury varying with age. Road traffic accidents and falls account for 80% of injuries

Effective management in the first 20 minutes after an accident can do much to reduce morbidity and mortality in children with trauma. In those who reach emergency facilities alive the commonest causes of preventable death are errors in the management of ventilation and circulation and failure to detect hidden injuries. Therefore early participation of senior staff who are familiar with the surgical, anaesthetic, and medical management of children is essential.

Because children are small multisystem injury is common. Thoracic and abdominal injuries are most commonly due to major blunt trauma, and, unlike in adults, it is unusual to see penetrating injuries. Furthermore, appreciable damage to internal organs can occur without overlying bony fractures. Associated head trauma is more common.

Duties of the paediatric trauma team

Team leader—Primary survey; secondary survey
Anaesthetist and nurse—Control of airway and ventilation; fluid balance; monitoring of central venous pressure (if needed)
Doctor and nurse—Establish intravenous access; blood sampling; procedures as required
Nurses—Pulse oximetry; electrocardiography; automatic recording of blood pressure; core temperature; measurement of patient from head to toe then estimation of age and weight

---

The assessment of children with multiple injuries should follow the same protocol outlined for adults. The tasks delineated in this chapter should be performed simultaneously by team members. The basic principle of resuscitation is to begin treatment of life threatening injuries immediately and not after complete evaluation of the child.

PRIMARY SURVEY

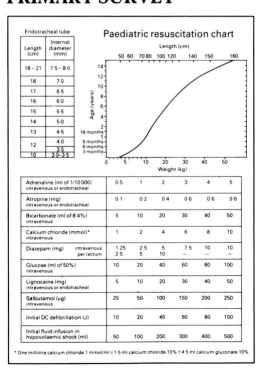

It is vital to know the weight of the child to calculate fluid volumes and drug doses. It is often impossible to weigh an injured child, but measuring head to toe length is easy, and reference to the nomogram on the paediatric resuscitation chart enables a reasonable estimate of age and weight.

Though efficient and aggressive management is essential, the conscious but injured child will be very frightened, and a team member should be allocated to give comfort and explain what is happening.

Airway management with protection of cervical spine

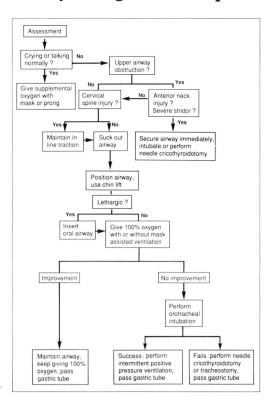

Children have specific anatomical differences compared with adults that can make maintenance of a clear airway and tracheal intubation difficult. They include:

- Large head relative to body size
- Small oral cavity with a relatively large tongue
- Large angle of the jaw (infant 140°, adult 120°)
- Epiglottis is more "U" shaped than in adults
- Larynx is cephalad (glottis at C3 in infant, C5-6 in adults) with an anterior and inferior inclination
- Cricoid ring is the narrowest part of the airway
- Trachea is short (newborn 4-5 cm, at 18 months 7-8 cm)
- Infants of 6 months or less are obligate nose breathers.

After assessment of the airway supplemental oxygen should be given to all children with trauma until further assessment shows that it is not required. Infants have a high oxygen consumption, a reduced functional residual capacity, and a high closing capacity, which leads to an increased right to left (physiological) shunt. This may be exacerbated, for example, by thoracic injury or diaphragmatic splinting due to raised intra-abdominal pressure. Nasal prongs are often better tolerated than masks by children younger than school age, but in the emergency setting they should be avoided in infants of less than six months, who are obligate nose breathers and in whom the prong may cause nasal obstruction.

If there is evidence of injury above the clavicles assume that the cervical spine has been damaged. A collar of appropriate size should be applied or, in infants, sandbags placed on either side of the head with tape across the forehead and on to a trolley to stop excessive head movement.

Clearing the airway

Secretions, vomit, blood, and foreign bodies in the airway should be removed. A free airway is best maintained in children by placing the head in slight extension and pulling the mandible forward, taking care not to place the supporting fingers in the submental triangle (any pressure in this area in children results in posterior displacement of the tongue and further airway obstruction). If the patient has a gag reflex he or she should be able to maintain an airway, and insertion of an artificial airway should not be attempted as it may precipitate choking, laryngospasm, or vomiting.

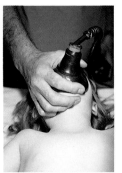 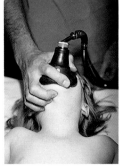

Maintaining a clear airway. (Left) Supporting fingers placed in the submental triangle causing posterior displacement of the tongue and airway obstruction. (Right) Correct placement of the hand and jaw lift.

Appropriate sizes and indications for use of paediatric equipment according to the age (approximate weight) of the child

Equipment	0-6 months (1-6 kg)	6-12 months (4-9 kg)	1-3 years (10-15 kg)	4-7 years (16-20 kg)	8-11 years (22-33 kg)
Airway/breathing:					
Oxygen facepiece	0	0/1	1	1/2	2/3 (Adult)
Oral airways	000/00	0/1	0/1	1/2	2
Resuscitator	Baby	Baby	Baby/adult	Adult	Adult
Breathing system	"T" piece	"T" piece	"T" piece	"T" piece	Coaxial
Laryngoscope	Straight blade	Straight blade	Child Macintosh	Child Macintosh	Adult Macintosh
Tracheal tubes (uncuffed)	2·5-3·5	3·5-4·0	4·0-5·0	5·0-6·0	5·5-7·0
Stylet	Small	Small	Small/meduum	Medium	Medium
Suction catheter (FG)	6	8	10-12	14	14
Circulation:					
Intravenous cannula (G)	24/22	22	22/18	20/16	18/14
Central venous pressure cannula (G)	20	20	18	18	16
Arterial cannula (G)	24/22	22	22	22	20
Ancillary equipment:					
Nasogastric tube (FG)	8	10	10-12	12	12-14
Chest drain (CH)	10-14	12-18	14-20	14-24	16-30
Urinary catheter (CH)	5 G Feeding tube	5 G Feeding tube/ Foley (8)	Foley (8)	Foley (10)	Foley (10-12)
Cervical collar			Small	Small	Medium

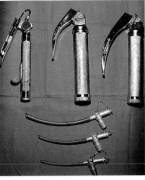

Laryngoscopes with orotracheal tubes fitted with Cardiff connecters. From left to right: Anderson-Magill, child Macintosh, and adult Macintosh.

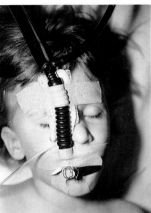

Correct fixation of Rees modified Ayres's "T" piece, endotracheal tube, and oral airway.

Artificial airway.

If there is no gag reflex or if there is any doubt as to the adequacy of the airway an artificial airway is required. A Guedel airway should be inserted and the chin supported as described above. If assisting ventilation the lungs should be gently inflated with 100% oxygen with pressures of <20 cm H_2O. Higher pressures cause gaseous distension of the stomach, thus increasing the risk of regurgitation and resulting in diaphragmatic splinting.

Tracheal intubation

Orotracheal intubation should be performed when hypoxia has been reversed by ventilation with a mask. **Do not persistently attempt to intubate the trachea of a hypoxic child without giving oxygen beforehand with a mask and airway.**

Laryngoscopes with straight blades should be used for children younger than 1 year (with the epiglottis being raised on the posterior surface); curved blades are satisfactory in older children. As a rough guide a tube of similar external diameter to the child's small finger or nostril is appropriate. Uncuffed endotracheal tubes must be used for all children who have not reached puberty, and there should be a small leak of gas around the tube as the lungs are inflated. If there is no leak the tube should be exchanged for the next smaller size. The orotracheal tube should be positioned such that 2-5 cm of it (according to age) are below the vocal cords. The tube lengths recommended in the paediatric resuscitation chart should result in an appropriate position. Inadvertent endobronchial intubation is a potential hazard, and auscultation in the axillae for bilateral breath sounds is essential. Firm fixation of both tube and breathing circuit is vital. For prolonged intubation (>1-2 hours) use plastic tracheal tubes.

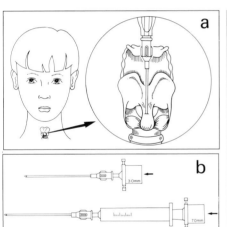

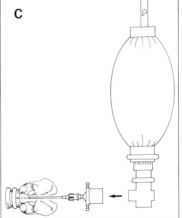

Technique for needle cricothyroidotomy. (a) The cricothyroid membrane is pierced at an angle of 45° by a 14 G cannula. Free aspiration of air confirms correct placement, and the cannula is advanced over the needle, which is then withdrawn; (b) a 3.0 mm endotracheal tube connecter fits into the female end of the intravenous cannula or a 7.0 mm connecter into the barrel of a 2 ml syringe; (c) the connecter is attached to the oxygen circuit.

Cricothyroidotomy

Needle cricothyroidotomy with a 14 G intravenous cannula is the preferred method of establishing airway access and control if bag and mask ventilation or intubation are unsuccessful. Tracheostomy should be undertaken only in controlled circumstances.

Gastric intubation

Acute gastric dilatation is commonly seen in the injured child. Almost all infants and children who are stressed swallow large quantities of air, and mask ventilation may add to this. Acute gastric dilatation may precipitate vomiting and aspiration, splint the diaphragm, and compress the inferior vena cava, diminishing venous return and thereby causing hypotension. A gastric tube must be passed in all injured children. If the cribriform plate is intact nasogastric intubation is the route of choice.

Breathing

Causes of inadequate ventilation

Bilateral
- Obstruction of upper respiratory tract
- Oesophageal intubation

Unilateral
- Pneumothorax
- Haemothorax
- Lung contusion
- Flail segment
- Bronchial rupture
- Foreign body in bronchus
- Rupture of diaphragm
- Endobronchial intubation

Ensure that both sides of the chest are being ventilated by inspection and auscultation. Look for central cyanosis and ensure that haemoglobin saturation measured with a pulse oximeter is above 90%. Count the respiratory rate, noting that normal values change with age.

Circulation and control of bleeding

Normal values for paediatric vital signs in patients who are not crying

Age	Heart rate (beats/min)	Blood pressure (systolic) (mm Hg)	Respiratory rate (breaths/min)	Blood volume (ml/kg)
<1 year	120-140	70-90	30-40	90
2-5 years	100-120	80-90	20-30	80
5-12 years	80-100	90-110	15-20	80

As in any victim of trauma major external haemorrhage must be controlled by direct pressure. The pulse rate and blood pressure are then recorded, the capillary refill time estimated, and the peripheral skin temperature and colour noted. Normal values for vital signs vary with age.

Advanced trauma life support classification of shock in children

	Class I <15%	Class II 20-25%	Class III 30-35%	Class IV 40%
Cardiovascular system (heart rate in beats/min)	Heart rate ↑ 10-20% Blood pressure normal	Tachycardia (>150) Systolic blood pressure ↓ Pulse pressure ↓	Tachycardia (>150) Systolic blood pressure ↓ ↓ Pulse pressure ↓ ↓	Tachycardia/ bradycardia Severe hypotension Peripheral pulses absent
Respiratory rate (breaths/min)	Normal	Tachypnoea (35-40)	Tachypnoea	Respiratory rate falls
Skin	Normal	Cool, peripheries cyanotic	Cold, clammy, cyanotic	Pale, cold
Central nervous system	Normal	Irritable, confused, aggressive	Lethargic	Comatose
Capillary refill time	Normal	Prolonged	Very prolonged	

A child's normal systolic blood pressure may be estimated by using the formula: blood pressure=80 mm Hg+(2×age). The increased physiological reserve of the child's circulation compared with that of adults means that vital signs may be only slightly abnormal despite considerable blood loss. Therefore the early diagnosis of impending shock in children is based on the appearance of the skin, the temperature of the extremities, the capillary refill time, and altered sensorium. The degree of shock, and hence blood loss, can be estimated from the classification of shock. Fluid resuscitation should not be withheld until vital signs are abnormal.

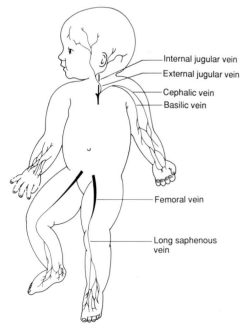

Appropriate vessels for intravenous cannulation.

Circulatory access

Venous access in hypovolaemic children with collapsed veins is difficult, especially in those less than 6 years old. Percutaneous cannulation of peripheral veins with an appropriately sized cannula should be attempted. In patients with appreciable abdominal injuries a vein draining to the superior vena cava should be chosen. If after two attempts access is not established the femoral or external jugular vein should be cannulated.

If all attempts at percutaneous cannulation fail a cut down should be undertaken in the median cephalic vein in the elbow or the long saphenous vein in the ankle.

In the interim intraosseous infusion is a useful method of emergency resuscitation in children. Crystalloids, colloids, and drugs can be given by this route, and the circulation time is usually less than 30 seconds. Cellulitis or osteomyelitis are potential complications.

The sites for intraosseous infusion are:
(1) The anterior tibial plateau 3 cm below the tibial tuberosity.
(2) The inferior one third of femur 3 cm above the external condyle.

Enter perpendicular to the bone (using a 16 G or 18 G bone marrow needle). Marrow aspiration indicates correct positioning.

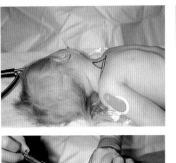
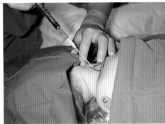
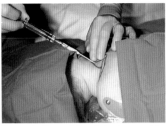
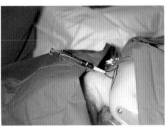

Cannulation of the right internal jugular vein.

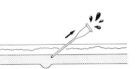

Transfix the vessel.

Withdraw the needle then the cannula until blood flows freely.

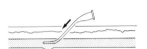

Advance the cannula into the vessel.

Technique for transfixion and cannulation of a peripheral artery.

Having established venous access take blood samples for determination of group and cross matching, full blood count, and urea and electrolyte concentrations.

Central venous cannulation in children is hazardous, especially if the patient is hypovolaemic, and should *never* be attempted by inexperienced doctors.

As in adults, a central venous pressure line is primarily for monitoring and not for giving fluids. Time must not be wasted inserting a central venous pressure line at the expense of other measures of basic life support during the initial resuscitation. Hypovolaemic children respond well to volume loading, allowing an adequate central venous pressure to be inferred from improvements in vital signs and skin perfusion.

When blood loss is massive (30-40%), however, intravascular volume must be assessed with a central venous pressure line.

The series of four pictures shows the procedure for cannulation of the right internal jugular vein. Tilt the patient's head downwards; extend the neck with a sandbag under the shoulder (there must be no suspicion of cervical spine injury); turn the head to the left and identify the triangle formed by the clavicle—the base—and the two heads of sternocleido-mastoid muscle (top left). With a strict aseptic technique pierce the skin at the apex of the triangle, aiming for the right nipple (top right). The internal jugular vein is very superficial and should be entered within 1-2 cm of the skin. Having punctured the vein, move the needle to a more horizontal position, then advance the cannula over the needle into the superior vena cava (bottom left). Withdraw the needle and ensure that blood can be aspirated freely (bottom right), then connect to a monitoring set.

Seriously injured patients should also have their intra-arterial pressure monitored. A transfixion technique is easiest in infants, and this should initially be attempted in the peripheral arteries.

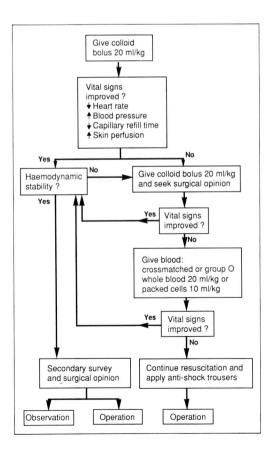

Fluid administration

Initial resuscitation should be with colloid (Haemaccel, Gelofusine, hetastarch, or 4·5% albumin (human plasma protein fraction). All fluids must be warmed to body temperature. An initial dose of 20 ml/kg should be given as a bolus, after which the response should be assessed and the decision tree followed. Patients with class III or IV shock require blood. If necessary blood that is not cross matched can be used; there is, however, usually time to get an immediate typed crossmatch that will eliminate serious reactions due to ABO incompatibility.

Whole blood, especially fresh whole blood, is rarely available. Red blood cells with a packed cell volume of 65-75% are often supplied. Administration of blood with a high packed cell volume is difficult through the small (22 G or 24 G) cannulas used in infants. Reconstitution of packed cells to a normal packed cell volume with human plasma protein fraction or fresh frozen plasma overcomes this problem but is time consuming.

Dysfunction and exposure

Paediatric Glasgow coma score

		>1 year	<1 year	
Eye opening	4	Spontaneously	Spontaneously	
	3	To verbal command	To shout	
	2	To pain	To pain	
	1	No response	No response	
Best motor response	5	Obeys commands		
	4	Localises pain	Localises pain	
	3	Flexion to pain	Flexion to pain	
	2	Extension to pain	Extension to pain	
	1	No response	No response	

		>5 years	2-5 years	0-2 years
Best verbal response	5	Oriented and converses	Appropriate words and phrases	Smiles and cries appropriately
	4	Disoriented and converses	Inappropriate words	Cries
	3	Inappropriate words	Cries	Inappropriate crying
	2	Incomprehensible sounds	Grunting	Grunting
	1	No response	No response	No response

Normal aggregate score:

<6 months	12
6-12 months	12
1-2 years	13
2-5 years	14
>5 years	14

Dysfunction

If the patient is old enough and well enough to cooperate the brain and spinal cord can be assessed rapidly by standard techniques. In young patients observation of motor function and ability to speak must suffice. An initial Glasgow coma scale score should be established.

Exposure

Removal of clothing is essential to allow adequate physical examination and facilitate practical procedures. Children, especially infants, however, lose heat rapidly as a result of their high ratio of surface area to weight, thin skin, and lack of subcutaneous tissue. Considerable heat loss may have occurred at the site of injury and during transportation. Monitoring temperature is a vital component of initial assessment. A fall in body temperature causes a rise in oxygen consumption as endogenous processes begin to increase heat production, peripheral vasoconstriction, and consequent lactic acidaemia. The ambient temperature of the resuscitation room should be raised and overhead heaters and warming blankets used. Plastic sheets can be used to cover exposed body parts.

SECONDARY SURVEY

Principles for the secondary survey

- Children should be assessed systematically according to a strict protocol
- Finding an injury should not stop the remainder of the evaluation
- Be gentle and pay particular attention to manipulation of the spinal cord axis
- Vital signs should be recorded repeatedly

After the primary survey, initial stabilisation of the cardiorespiratory system, and treatment of shock a complete physical examination takes place.

Head and neck

Causes of secondary brain damage

Hypoxia

—Respiratory insufficiency

Cerebral ischaemia

—Systemic hypotension

—Fall in cerebral perfusion pressure secondary to raised intracranial pressure from cerebral oedema or an intracranial mass lesion

Ages at which acute subdural and extradural haematomas are usually seen in children and associated incidences of seizures and skull fractures

	Acute subdural haematomas	Extradural haematomas
Age at which usually seen	<12 months	>2 years
Associated incidence of seizures	High (75%)	Low (<25%)
Associated incidence of skull fractures	Low (30%)	High (75%)

As in adult patients fully examine the head for lacerations; the skull for fractures; the eyes for injury (also remember penetrating injury) and pupillary function; the ears and nose for leakage of cerebrospinal fluid; the face for fractures and lacerations; the mouth for loose teeth; and, finally, the neck for cervical displacement. Frequent assessment of the Glasgow coma score is essential.

Primary brain damage that occurs at the time of the injury cannot be reversed. Secondary brain damage occurs as a result of cerebral hypoxia or ischaemia and can be minimised by maintaining oxygenation and an adequate cerebral perfusion pressure.

A child's brain is vulnerable to accelerative, decelerative, and shear forces, which result in focal intracranial mass lesions (cerebral contusions, lacerations, haemorrhages, and oedema). Raised intracranial presure secondary to diffuse cerebral swelling is the most common cause of death in children with head injuries.

Acute subdural haematomas are often bilateral and are associated with a high incidence of seizures and a low incidence of skull fractures. If there is no history of appreciable trauma the possibility of non-accidental injury should be considered.

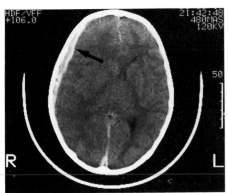

Computed tomogram showing right subdural haematoma.

Initial management of severe head injury

- Restoration of the circulating blood volume
- Tracheal intubation
- Adequate oxygenation ($S_aO_2 > 90\%$)
- Hyperventilation (P_aCO_2 3·5-4·0 kPa)
- Administration of mannitol 0·5-1·0 g/kg

Criteria for skull radiography after head injury in children

- Age <1 year
- Loss of consciousness ≥5 minutes
- Lethargy, coma, or stupor
- Focal neurological signs
- Skull penetration
- Skull depression
- Palpable scalp haematoma
- Cerebrospinal fluid from nose or ear
- Blood in middle ear
- Battle's sign
- Racoon eyes

Neck and spine

Confusing radiological features of children's cervical spines

Growth centres resemble fractures
- Cartilaginous plate at the base of the odontoid (closes at between 3 and 5 years)
- Secondary ossification centre at apex of odontoid (present from 2-12 years)
- Secondary ossification centre at tip of spinous processes

Pseudosubluxation
- Anterior displacement of C2 on C3 (30% of children <7 years). Much less commonly C3 on C4. Perform radiography in neutral and extension positions if clinically safe

Hypermobility
- Increased distance between dens and anterior arch of C1 (15% of children <5 years)

Paediatric trauma

Extradural haematomas are most often unilateral and associated with a high incidence of skull fractures and a low incidence of seizures. The biphasic presentation of extradural haematomas ("lucid interval") is less common in children.

About 75% of skull fractures are linear, but they may be depressed, compound, or basal, and in children of less than 3 years, the cranial sutures can undergo traumatic separation (diasteal fractures).

The clinical manifestations of raised intracranial pressure or skull fractures are the same in children as in adults. Infants with open fontanelles and mobile sutures, however, are more tolerant to an expanding intracranial mass, although when decompensation does occur it is rapid and often irrecoverable. A bulging fontanelle or sutural diastases in an infant implies serious cerebral trauma.

As in adults an initial Glasgow coma score of <7 or a declining score are indications for immediate aggressive management. In particular, restoration of the circulating volume is vital and should not be limited by considerations of fluid restriction to control cerebral oedema. A neurosurgical opinion should be sought urgently, and if the patient is haemodynamically stable computed tomography should be performed immediately.

In children, head injury alone does not usually produce shock and hypotension due to hypovolaemia; most bleeding usually occurs elsewhere in the body. Extensive scalp lacerations, however, may bleed sufficiently to cause hypovolaemic shock, and in small infants intracranial haemorrhage may be enough to cause hypovolaemia.

After head injury vomiting and seizures are more common in children than in adults. Both symptoms tend to be self limiting, but if either persists a serious head injury should be suspected. Repeated seizures cause an increase in intracranial pressure by increasing cerebral blood flow, and anticonvulsants should be given. Intravenous diazepam 0·15-0·25 mg/kg is the drug of first choice; this may cause respiratory depression, so be prepared to provide artificial ventilation. Follow this with phenytoin 15-20 mg/kg by slow intravenous injection (1-2 mg/kg/min); monitor the electrocardiogram continuously during the injection.

Minor head injury is extremely common in children; the overwhelming majority of children with such injury do not develop intracranial pathology and the need for radiography is often questionable.

Spinal cord injuries are rare in children, constituting only 5% of all spinal cord trauma. But there should be a high index of suspicion in any child with major trauma, especially if he or she has an appreciable head injury.

Careful clinical and radiological examination should be undertaken (see previous articles on spinal cord trauma). Assessing paralysis and altered sensation, however, can be very difficult, especially in infants. Mass flexion withdrawal in response to stimulation may be indistinguishable from normal withdrawal in this age group. Furthermore, 50% of children with serious spinal injuries have normal radiographs, and radiological normality should not deter a clinical diagnosis of spinal injury. Conversely, there are several peculiarities in radiographs of the immature spine that may lead to overdiagnosis of spinal injury.

Thorax

Occult chest injuries in children
- Pulmonary contusion
- Pulmonary laceration
- Intrapulmonary haemorrhage
- Tracheobronchial tear
- Myocardial contusion
- Diaphragmatic rupture
- Partial aortic or other great vessel disruption
- Oesophageal tears

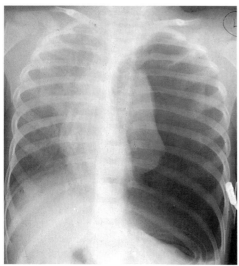

Radiograph of left tension pneumothorax causing deviation of the mediastinum to the right.

Blunt chest trauma is common in children whereas penetrating injury is rare; but the approach to diagnosis and management is the same as in adults. About 15-20% of children with major injuries have chest trauma that requires immediate management. Early diagnosis is essential: of the children who die of chest injury more than 90% die in the first few hours after the accident. The vast majority of thoracic injuries (85-90%) can be managed by standard procedures. Remember that patients with thoracic trauma have a high incidence of associated injuries (>50%), most commonly of the head, abdomen, or an extremity.

The chest wall should be examined for bruising, wounds, and asymmetry of movement. The high compliance of a child's chest wall, however, allows ready transfer of energy to intrathoracic structures, and appreciable organ damage may be present with minimal evidence of chest wall injury.

The mobility of mediastinal structures in children means that there is a lower incidence of injury to the airway and great blood vessels than in adults, but cardiovascular and ventilatory compromise occur readily as a result of trauma causing mediastinal shift.

If a pneumothorax (indicated by inequality of air entry) is under tension it requires immediate drainage. Open pneumothorax is unusual in children. Flail segments are also uncommon in children but require early treatment with chest drainage, intermittent positive pressure ventilation, and positive end expiratory pressure. Haemoptysis, subcutaneous emphysema, and a persistent air leak after drainage of a pneumothorax all suggest underlying lung damage.

Patients with pulmonary contusion present with tachypnoea, breathlessness, and hypoxia. The symptoms are often exacerbated by inhalation of gastric contents, especially if the abdomen has been compressed. If the child has undergone a garrotting injury tracheal rupture should be suspected, especially if there is subcutaneous emphysema in the neck. Noisy breathing and a persistent leak through the chest drain suggest a tracheal or major bronchial tear. As in adults diaphragmatic rupture, most commonly on the left side, is often missed clinically but should be suspected if the left side of the diaphragm is not clearly visualised in the chest radiograph.

Heart and great blood vessels

Arrhythmias are unusual in children with trauma and if present suggest myocardial injury

Myocardial contusion is rare in children but is suggested by arrhythmias in a child who has sustained blunt trauma to the anterior chest wall. Continuous electrocardiography is vital. Cardiac tamponade due to haemopericardium is also rare because penetrating injury is unusual in children. The signs are the same as in adults, and drainage using a 14 G intravenous cannula should be by the left subxiphoid route. Aortic rupture occurs most commonly at the origin of the left subclavian artery. A widened mediastinum, fractures of the first or second ribs, and obliteration of the aortic knuckle are suggestive signs in the chest radiograph.

Clinical assessment of the signs of hypovolaemic shock should be frequently repeated to assess the response to fluid resuscitation.

Abdomen

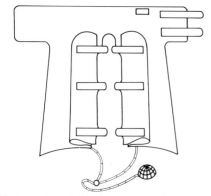

Pneumatic anti-shock trousers will maintain central circulating volume during fluid resuscitation.

The basic principle governing the evaluation of a child with a possible abdominal injury is to determine whether an operation is necessary either for an acute abdomen or for controlling haemorrhage.

As in thoracic injuries blunt trauma is most common. Penetrating wounds are rare but, when present, require an operation. If haemorrhage is substantial and rapid the use of pneumatic anti-shock trousers may be life saving, providing time for resuscitation and exploring the abdomen.

Abdominal injuries caused by rapid deceleration forces

Duodenal
    —Perforation
    —Obstructing haematoma

Pancreatic
Rupture of hollow viscera
    —At the ligament of Treitz
    —Near the ileocaecal valve

Mesenteric avulsion
Renal
    —Vascular
    —Parenchymal
    —Collecting system

Bladder

Early passage of a nasogastric tube of appropriate size is essential in children. Careful and gentle clinical examination of the conscious child will produce evidence of appreciable abdominal injury, which may be present despite minimal indications of trauma in the abdominal wall. The pattern and methods of clinical examination are the same as in adults.

As in adults the spleen and liver are the most commonly injured solid organs, but rapid deceleration forces cause abdominal compression and may result in other injuries. A renal injury should be suspected in every child with tenderness of the flank and red blood cells in the urine. The lumbar spine, ribs, and pelvis are also commonly injured.

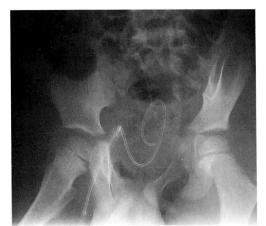

Radiograph showing fractured pelvis caused by a crush injury. A suprapubic catheter is in situ.

Assessment of the abdomen may be difficult in an unconscious child. Haemodynamic instability or questionable abdominal findings are indications for computed tomography. Also, if the patient receives general anaesthesia for other surgery lavage can help to determine whether abdominal exploration is required. A paediatric size peritoneal dialysis catheter is inserted through the lower abdominal midline under direct vision, remembering that a child's abdominal wall is much thinner than an adult's. Then 10 ml/kg of Ringer-lactate solution (1000 ml maximum dose) is run in over 10 minutes. Lavage results in peritoneal irritation for up to 48 hours, making subsequent assessment difficult. In practice it is much less often needed in children than in adults and a decision to perform lavage should not be undertaken lightly.

The rate of urine output must be measured through a catheter in children with trauma, unless they can void spontaneously. The approach (through the urethra or suprapubic) is determined by the clinical evidence of urethral injury. Urine should always be dipstick tested for blood, glucose, etc.

All children with multiple injuries should undergo cervical spine, chest, and pelvic radiography. If damage to the urinary tract is suspected a one shot intravenous pyelogram in the resuscitation room can often provide useful information in patients who require urgent abdominal exploration. Many North American centres advocate thoracic and abdominal computed tomography for investigating children with multiple injuries, provided that they are haemodynamically stable.

Skeletal and soft tissue injuries

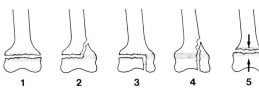

  1   2   3   4   5

The Salter-Harris classification of physeal fractures.

The principles of management of skeletal and soft tissue damage are the same as those for adults. In children the history of the injury is important. The radiological diagnosis of skeletal injury around the joints is more difficult in children because of the growth plate and lack of mineralisation of the epiphysis. Radiographs of the opposite side (if uninjured) may be helpful.

The pattern of fractures is different in children. They may be through the growth plate (Salter-Harris classification[1] types I-V), greenstick (only through one cortex of a long bone), or buckle (bony angulation without a fracture). Because of potential arresting of growth, malalignment of joints, and traumatic arthritis it is important to recognise fractures through the epiphysis. Supracondylar fractures at the elbow have a high incidence of associated vascular injury. Old healed fractures should alert the medical team to the possibility of non-accidental injury. The proportional blood loss after pelvic or long bone fractures in children is greater and may be an important cause of initial haemodynamic instability.

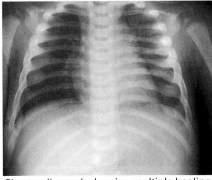

Chest radiograph showing multiple healing rib fractures after non-accidental injury.

Paediatric trauma
Burns

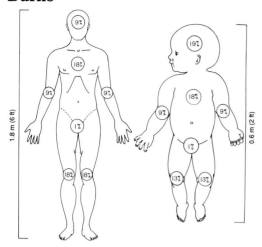

Body surface area in adults and children.

Scalds from hot water are the most common cause of burns in children, and management does not differ appreciably from that of adult patients (see chapter on burns). The change in body proportions as children grow means that calculation of the percentage total body surface area burnt cannot be based on the adult "rule of nines." Accurate estimation of the percentage of the total body surface area burnt requires the use of detailed charts.[2]

Non-accidental injury

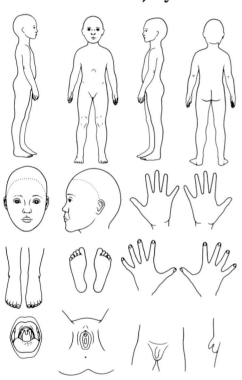

Diagram used for precise marking of injuries in a suspected case of non-accidental injury.

A wide variety of injuries can be caused by physical child abuse. Various points in the history and examination should suggest the possibility of non-accidental injury. Initial resuscitation and management of the battered child are the prime responsibilities of the casualty medical team, but the need to inform the appropriate authorities must not be overlooked. Careful recording of injuries is vital, and standard diagrams should be available for this purpose.

Diagnostic criteria for non-accidental injury

- Delay in seeking medical advice
- Account of the accident is vague and inconsistent among parties
- Discrepancy between the history and the degree of injury
- Parental behaviour is abnormal, lack of concern for their child
- Interaction between child and parents is abnormal
- Finger tip bruising, especially over upper arms, trunk, sides of face, ears, or neck
- Bizarre injuries—for example, bites, cigarette burns, or rope marks
- Sharply demarcated burns in unusual areas
- Perioral injuries—for example, torn frenulum
- Retinal haemorrhage
- Multiple subdural haemorrhages
- Ruptured internal organs without a history of major trauma
- Perianal or genital injury
- Long bone fractures in children <3 years
- Previous injuries—for example, old scars, healing fractures

---

Pain relief

Control of pain

- After resuscitation give morphine 25 µg/kg intravenously
- Titrate further doses of 10 µg/kg against patient's response
- Do not give narcotic drugs to patients with head injuries

Adequate control of pain is humane and will improve a child's cooperation with diagnosis, investigation, and management of the injury. After initial fluid resuscitation a bolus of 25 µg/kg of morphine should be given intravenously. Further doses may be given at 10 minute intervals, titrated against the patient's response to just control pain. **Patients with appreciable head injuries whose conscious level is depressed or fluctuating should not receive opioid analgesics.**

Throughout the period of the secondary survey the child's response to resuscitation and general condition should be constantly reassessed. Subsequent management depends on the expertise and facilities of the receiving hospital. If the anaesthetic, surgical, and intensive care services are not suited to children a protocol for transfer to a designated paediatric centre should be an important part of the initial evaluation and management.

The paediatric resuscitation chart is reproduced from the paper by P A Oakley (*BMJ* 1988;**297**:817-9) and was devised from the guidelines of the Resuscitation Council (UK). The line drawings were prepared by the department of education medical illustration services, St Bartholomew's Hospital, London. The radiographs were kindly provided by Drs B Kendall, D Shaw, C Hall, and D Hatch, Hospital for Sick Children, Great Ormond Street, London.

1 Salter RB, Harris WR. Injuries involving the epiphyseal plate. *American Journal of Bone and Joint Surgery* 1963;**45**:587-622.
2 Lund CC, Bowder NC. The estimation of area of burns. *Surg Gynecol Obstet* 1944;**79**:353-60.

MANAGEMENT OF SEVERE BURNS

Colin Robertson, Oliver Fenton

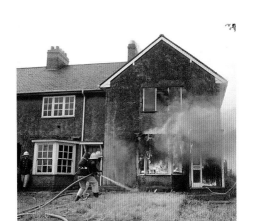

At the scene of a fire first aid procedures are often life saving. Medical staff should use the following instructions for preparing a victim for evacuation to a hospital.

Under the direction of the fire service and ensuring the safety of the rescuers the patient should be removed from the scene of injury to a place of safety and fresh air.

Flames and heat track upwards, so the patient should be kept supine and rolled or covered with a heavy blanket, coat, or rug to extinguish any residual flames. Take care not to get burnt yourself, especially if dealing with petrol burns or self immolation.

If the clothing is still smouldering or hot apply large amounts of cold water. Clothing saturated with boiling liquids or steam should be removed rapidly, but do not remove burnt clothing that is adherent to the skin. Cover burnt areas with clean (sterile if available) towels or sheets and ensure that the patient is kept warm. Do not apply wet soaks or ice packs or use them during transit as this will not provide any pain relief for patients with full thickness burns and can cause profound hypothermia, especially in children.

Evacuate the patient to the receiving hospital as quickly as possible. In patients with severe burns or those who have been exposed to smoke or fumes high flow oxygen through a facemask should be given during transit.

Alert the receiving accident and emergency department by radio or telephone as to the number and ages of the patients and the severity of their burns, together with the estimated time of arrival.

Reception and resuscitation

> **Necessary information on incident**
>
> - Its nature (house fire, blast, release of steam or hot gas, etc)
> - If possible, the nature of burning materials (furniture, polyurethane foam, polyvinyl chloride, etc)
> - Was there any explosion?
> - Was the patient in an enclosed space?
> - For how long was the patient exposed to smoke or fire?
> - The time elapsed from burn/injury/smoke inhalation to arrival in hospital.

The primary assessment, investigation, and treatment of a patient with severe burns should be a continuous and integrated process rather than a stepwise progression. While assessment is being performed a member of staff must obtain the necessary information about the incident from the ambulance crew and other emergency services. This should then be conveyed to the senior doctor in charge of the patient.

Management of the airway

> **Clinical features indicating smoke or thermal injury to respiratory tract**
>
> Altered consciousness
>
> Direct burns to face or oropharynx
>
> Hoarseness, stridor
>
> Soot in nostrils or sputum
>
> Expiratory rhonchi
>
> Dysphagia

Rapidly examine the patient for clinical evidence of smoke inhalation and thermal injury to the respiratory tract. In patients with one or more of the features described in the box respiratory obstruction from pharyngeal or laryngeal oedema may develop rapidly. In such patients early endotracheal intubation performed by an experienced doctor is essential. Mucosal swelling of the oropharynx and epiglottis can be extremely rapid, and delay can render tracheostomy necessary. In patients in whom complete respiratory obstruction has already occurred or intubation is unsuccessful, or both, immediate cricothyrotomy or "mini" tracheostomy is required, followed by formal tracheostomy. It should be emphasised, however, that in patients with severe burns the tracheostomy site is an important site of infection.

Management of severe burns

Immediate investigations

- Peak expiratory flow rate (if possible)
- Arterial blood gas tensions
- Carboxyhaemoglobin concentration
- Blood grouping and cross matching
- Packed cell volume
- Urea and electrolyte concentrations
- 12 Lead electrocardiography
- Chest radiography

All patients suspected of having inhaled smoke should be given humidified high flow oxygen (an inspired oxygen concentration (F_{iO_2}) of 40-60%) through a face mask. If bronchospasm is present give the patient a β_2 agonist (such as salbutamol or terbutaline) with an oxygen powered nebuliser.

Frequent repeated clinical assessment of the airway and ventilation is mandatory in patients with all types of injuries caused by fire, together with further measurements of arterial blood gas tensions, carboxyhaemoglobin concentration and, if the patient can comply, peak expiratory flow rates.

Intravenous access

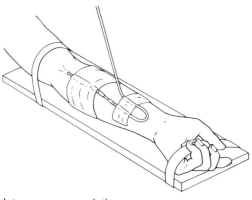

Intravenous cannulation.

Establishing adequate intravenous access must not be delayed. Insert and secure one or more large bore (needle gauge 14-16) intravenous cannulas. If possible use 10-15 cm cannulas to reduce the risk of dislodgement. The normal and easiest sites for percutaneous insertion of intravenous cannulas are the forearms and antecubital fossae. Narrow bore cannulas inserted into small veins on the back of the hands are of little practical value. Occasionally, alternative sites such as the external jugular and femoral veins or the long saphenous vein at the ankle must be used, although the saphenous vein is prone to early occlusion.

Intravenous cutdown in the cubital fossae or on the long saphenous vein in the groin may be required if percutaneous intravenous access cannot be performed. This approach can be made through burnt skin, but if this is the case do not attempt to suture the resulting gaping wound. If possible, before attaching the tubing of the intravenous drip take enough blood through the cannula for cross matching and determining blood group, packed cell volume, and urea and electrolyte concentrations.

Intravenous fluid requirements

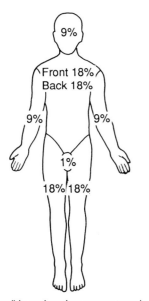

"Rule of nine" in estimating percentage body surface area.

For rapid assessment the "rule of nine" is useful. Do not include areas of simple erythema in the estimate. The size of small burns can be judged roughly by considering the palmar surface of the patient's closed hand as about 1% of the total body surface area. Use your own hand to map out the burnt area, and then make allowances for the size of your hand compared with the patient's—for example, it would be three times the size of a 1 year old child's and twice the size of a 5 year old child's. The result can be cross checked by mapping the size of the unburnt area. In patients with very large burns it is simpler to measure the unburnt area and then subtract from 100.

Example of how to judge the volume required for intravenous replacement

Weight of patient who has sustained a burn= 70 kg

Body surface area covered=35%

Volume of colloid required in first four hours after injury=$\dfrac{35 \times 70}{2}$

=1225 ml

Start treatment with intravenous fluids; the first 500 ml should be 0·9% saline. If colloid is then used—for example, 5% albumin, Polygelatine, or Dextran 70—the volume of fluid required for intravenous replacement treatment for the first four hours since injury should be judged roughly as the percentage of the body surface area of the burn multiplied by the body weight (kg) divided by two. If crystalloid alone is used this volume should be doubled.

Patients with full thickness burns that cover >10% of the body surface area may require a transfusion of red blood cells in addition to fluid replacement.

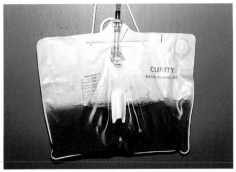

Urine from a patient with electrical burns indicates haemoglobinuria.

Insert a urinary catheter and start hourly measurements of urine volume. Note the colour and consistency of the initial urine in patients with severe flame or high voltage electrical burns. The urine may be a treacly black, indicating haemoglobinuria or myoglobinuria, or both. This is of prognostic importance for subsequent renal function.

In elderly patients, patients with cardiorespiratory disease, and patients who have delayed presentation consider inserting a central venous pressure line if you are experienced in the technique. This can play an important part in the subsequent restoration of volume in a patient with a severe burn. The risks of infection related to a central line are small in the early stages. With current methods of line management these risks are outweighed by the importance of the line for monitoring and access.

Analgesia and reassurance

Pain relief in patients with severe burns

Entonox—for conscious, cooperative patients, especially in the prehospital phase

Opioids—give intravenously in small aliquots titrated to the patient's clinical response

Severe burns cause both pain and distress. Analgesia and reassurance should be given as soon as possible. Treatment for pain in patients with severe burns must be tailored to the patient's individual requirements. Full thickness burns, if present, are pain free, but all patients will be frightened and distressed, and constant reassurance and communication are vital.

A mixture of 50% nitrous oxide and 50% oxygen (Entonox) given by an on demand system with a tight fitting facemask can provide simple and effective analgesia, particularly before arrival in hospital. Subsequently, if required, an opioid such as Cyclimorph (cyclizine and morphine) should be given intravenously in aliquots of 1 mg at a dose carefully titrated to the clinical response.

Reassessment

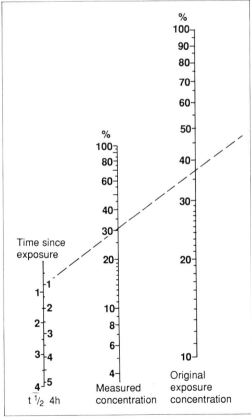

Nomogram for calculating carboxyhaemoglobin concentration at time of exposure.

Time since exposure is given in two scales to allow for effects of previous oxygen administration as half life of carboxyhaemoglobin (left scale assumes a half life of 3 h).

The airway

Confirm that the patient's airway is secure and that ventilation is adequate. Repeat the measurements of arterial blood gas tensions and the analysis of carboxyhaemoglobin concentrations, which give an approximate guide to the amount of smoke inhaled; concentrations at the time of exposure can be predicted by using the nomogram. For example, if the carboxyhaemoglobin concentration is 30% one hour after exposure the concentration at exposure would have been about 37%.

Clinical features of carbon monoxide poisoning correlate only moderately well with carboxyhaemoglobin concentrations. The so called "classic" feature of cherry red mucous membranes is a rarely seen, totally unreliable clinical sign.

Other toxic gases, such as hydrogen cyanide, hydrogen sulphide, and hydrogen chloride, are often produced in fires. They may cause local irritation to both upper and lower airways as well as acting systemically as direct cellular poisons. The possibility of cyanide poisoning should be considered in patients with high carboxyhaemoglobin concentrations who are apnoeic and have metabolic acidosis. In these patients emergency resuscitation with assisted ventilation is required, and the use of cyanide antidotes (such as sodium thiosulphate with amyl nitrite (for enhanced distribution), and dicobalt edetate) should be considered.

Ensure that deep circumferential burns of the thorax are not causing restriction in chest expansion and hence ventilation (see below).

Management of severe burns

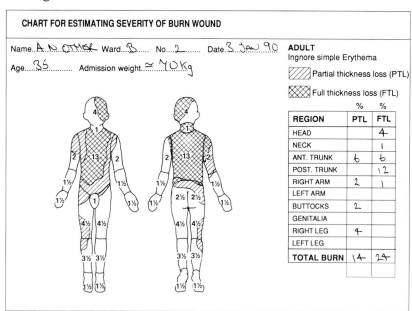

CHART FOR ESTIMATING SEVERITY OF BURN WOUND

Name..A. N. OTHER.... Ward...B..... No...2..... Date..3 Jan 90

Age.....35......   Admission weight. ≃ 70 Kg

ADULT
Ingnore simple Erythema

▨ Partial thickness loss (PTL)

▩ Full thickness loss (FTL)

REGION	PTL %	FTL %
HEAD		4
NECK		1
ANT. TRUNK	6	6
POST. TRUNK		12
RIGHT ARM	2	1
LEFT ARM		
BUTTOCKS	2	
GENITALIA		
RIGHT LEG	4	
LEFT LEG		
TOTAL BURN	14	24

Lund and Browder chart.

Treatment with fluids

The rule of nine, which is used in the rapid assessment of the burn injury, can result in overestimation of the extent of the burn. More accurate assessment can be made with Lund and Browder charts and the rate of intravenous replacement adjusted accordingly.

Formulas for intravenous fluid requirements are, however, only rough guides and need modification according to the patient's clinical state. Regular checks and recording of pulse rate, blood pressure, central venous pressure (if indicated), urine output, packed cell volume, and peripheral perfusion and of the trends in their values can provide additional guidance for adjusting the rate of infusion.

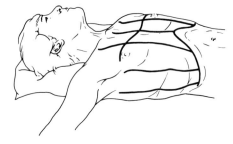

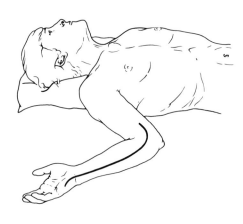

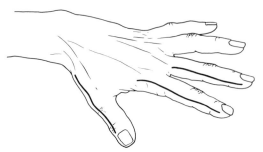

Escharotomy of the chest, arm, and fingers.

The burns

Pending the patient's transfer from the accident and emergency department to the ward or specialist burns unit the burnt area should be covered with a sterile, warm, non-adherent dressing. A layer of Clingfilm covered by a dry sheet and blanket is effective. Under no circumstances should a patient be transferred in wet sheets or towels as this can lead to hypothermia, with occasional fatal consequences.

Deep circumferential burns over the limbs, neck, and chest can produce a tourniquet like effect as the damaged skin is unable to expand as tissue oedema develops. If this occurs escharotomies (longitudinal incisions of the skin) are required to permit adequate circulation. It may be necessary to perform these before transfer. The affected part should be incised under sterile conditions on both sides in much the same way as a plaster of Paris cast is bivalved. Ensure that the entire length of the constriction is released and take the incisions right to the tips of affected digits.

If escharotomy of the chest is required vertical incisions along anterior and posterior axillary lines should be made. If sufficient chest expansion does not occur further incisions in the midline and midclavicular lines and tranverse incisions may be required. Escharotomy does not require anaesthesia as the burns are full thickness burns. If it does cause pain then escharotomy is probably not indicated.

Failure to perform an early escharotomy can lead to the loss of a limb; therefore if doubtful always err on the side of escharotomy. The incisions do not cause any additional scarring as the burns are full thickness ones. Substantial bleeding occurs from the wounds, and sterile absorbent dressings should be applied and, if necessary, blood replacement given. Ensure that the patient is adequately protected against tetanus.

Lethal burns

Few patients survive full thickness burns that cover more than 70% of the body surface area. As a very rough guide, if the patient's age added to the percentage of the body surface area of the burn exceeds 100 the chances of survival are low. Any decision not to treat a patient with a lethal burn aggressively must be taken by a consultant with experience in burns. If aggressive resuscitation is not to be instituted in a patient the other aspects of reassurance and analgesia are of even greater importance. Remember that even patients with 100% full thickness burns are usually conscious and sentient.

Information required by burns unit

- Name, age, and sex of patient
- Percentage of body surface area covered by and depth of burns
- Involvement of "special" areas such as the face, head, and perineum
- Time of injury
- Presence of respiratory problems
- Treatment instituted and response

The photograph of a burning house was supplied by the Royal Society for Prevention of Accident and that depicting haemoglobulinuria was reproduced from the advanced trauma life support™ (ATLS™) slide set by kind permission of the American College of Surgeons' committee on trauma. The nomogram was reproduced with kind permission from the paper by C J Clark *et al* (*Lancet* 1981;i:1332-5), and the drawings depicting intravenous access and escharotomy were prepared by the education and medical illustration services department, St Bartholomew's Hospital.

General aspects

Ask the patient and the relatives about pre-existing medical conditions, especially if these may be relevant to the therapeutic intervention being performed—for example, obstructive airways disease and ischaemic heart disease. Consider the possibility of underlying medical conditions that may have led to the burn injury—for example, epilepsy, a cerebrovascular episode, hypoglycaemia, drug or alcohol overdose.

In elderly patients, patients with known ischaemic heart disease, and all patients with a carboxyhaemoglobin concentration >15% obtain a 12 lead electrocardiogram and attach a cardiac monitor. Myocardial ischaemia or infarction and arrhythmias occur commonly and often do not have their usual clinical features.

Consider the possibility of non-accidental injury in children.

Do not give prophylaxis with antibiotics or steroids.

Depending on local policies discuss the patient's management with the burns or plastic surgical receiving team. If the patient is being transported within the hospital or to another referral hospital adequate intravenous fluids and analgesics should be transported along with him or her. All patients suspected of having inhaled smoke or requiring additional care of the airway must be escorted by an experienced anaesthetist with appropriate equipment.

Make clear, concise notes, which must accompany the patient and should include the size of the burn; the weight of the patient; the time when intravenous fluids were started; which drugs were given for pain relief and at what dose and time they were given; the urine and fluids chart; and details of special problems.

BLAST AND GUNSHOT INJURIES

Ian Haywood, David Skinner

The incidence of blast and gunshot injuries is increasing throughout the world. This article deals with management problems that are specific to these injuries.

Doctors and nurses treating patients who have blast or gunshot injuries should remember that in nearly all cases there will be forensic or medicolegal consequences and that, although patient care is of prime importance, they have certain duties to record information with these consequences in mind. Such information may be required in subsequent legal prosecution or to help the victims to obtain adequate compensation. Accurate record keeping with retention of a personal copy for the long term is important.

The early management of patients who have suffered bomb blast or gunshot injuries is the same as for those with other injuries, and the patient should be managed with the same systematic approach in the primary and secondary surveys and definitive management. Certain specific actions must be taken, however, because of the mechanism of injury.

Injuries caused by explosions

Blast injuries are caused by → Shock waves
↘ Blast winds

Blunt trauma, especially to the head, is common in people injured as a consequence of an explosion. It may be due to either translocation or a phenomenon such as the collapse of a building.

Flash burns may occur, or more serious burns, with the risk of smoke inhalation, may follow secondary conflagration. These injuries are managed as described in the article in this series on major burns.

The specific injuries caused by explosions may be those due to blast or penetrating missiles, or both, set in motion by the explosion. Blast injuries may be caused by either shock waves or columns of air set in motion by the explosion, which are known as blast winds.

A shock wave is a front of high pressure travelling at just over the speed of sound. When reflected by solid objects it may be multiplied severalfold. The circumstance in which injury occurs is therefore of prime importance—that is, the severity of injury is likely to be increased in victims of explosions in enclosed spaces or water.

A blast wind follows the shock wave caused by an explosion and consists of rapidly moving air, which may cause injuries as it may carry fragments of materials such as glass and metal.

The mechanism by which shock waves damage the body is multifactorial. Clinically, the shock wave produces tissue damage mainly at gas-tissue interfaces, and, therefore, serious lesions tend to be found in the upper and lower respiratory tracts and the abdomen. In the nasal air passages there may be damage to the olfactory nerve endings, producing anosmia. The tympanic membranes may be ruptured: this is a useful clinical indicator that exposure to significant blast has occurred, but as blast waves may be unpredictable the converse does not necessarily hold.

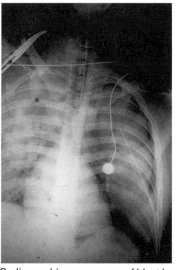

Radiographic appearance of blast lung a few hours after injury.

Lung damage presents clinically in two ways

(1) As a sudden severe massive contusion producing instant, usually fatal, respiratory failure

(2) Diffuse lung damage may develop, the onset of which may be delayed for up to 48 hours. Such damage, from which survival is possible, may occur in up to 5% of those injured by explosions. The clinical presentation is similar to that of the adult respiratory distress syndrome, with increasing respiratory failure and radio-opacity of lung fields, but is coupled in some cases with air entering the circulation, producing small arterial air emboli, which in turn may produce secondary damage. Air may continue to enter the circulation for some time after exposure to a blast, and the risk is theoretically increased with positive pressure ventilation. Intermittent positive pressure respiration and, more definitely, positive end expiratory pressure should therefore be avoided if possible. Diagnosis may sometimes be confirmed by the presence of air in the retinal vessels. Clinically, central nervous system damage may become apparent. Pneumothoraces, with or without tension, can occur. Deterioration may be precipitated by any form of exercise, however mild.

Massive damage to major abdominal organs occurs but is rarely seen in those who survive blast injuries. The common intra-abdominal injuries in survivors are multiple contusions with haemorrhage in the subserous, intramuscular, and submucosal planes of the viscera. Acute intestinal perforation may occur, but more commonly this is delayed for as long as five days. Such perforation is due to necrosis secondary to ischaemia at the site of the haematomas. There may be diffuse abdominal pain and tenderness, but, because there inevitably is concomitant pulmonary injury, with its associated anaesthetic risk, laparotomy should be reserved for those patients in whom there is clear evidence of perforation—that is, localised peritonitis or free air on radiography.

Management of blast injuries

(1) Thorough examination includes:
- Chest—examine for signs of respiratory failure and pneumothorax —perform chest radiography to exclude pneumothorax: examine baseline appearance of lung fields, for signs of the adult respiratory distress syndrome, and for free gas under the diaphragm
- Abdomen—examine for local peritonitis and bowel sounds
- Central nervous system—examine for abnormal signs
- Funduscopy for air emboli
- External auditory meati for perforated tympanic membranes
- Olfactory function (for medicolegal compensation)

(2) Treatment. Confine patient to a chair or bed to prevent exertion
- Give oxygen by mask
- Maintain ventilation if there is respiratory failure, but balance against the risk of embolism
- If intermittent positive pressure respiration is elected consider prophylactic chest drains
- Treat other injuries as necessary
- Perform laparotomy in cases of definite perforation

(3) If exposed to appreciable blast, **even if no injury is apparent**, observe patient for 48 hours

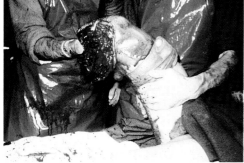
Traumatic amputation caused by blast winds.

Blast winds

Blast winds are responsible for the severe disintegration and dismemberment caused by explosions, but these are usually fatal. Occasionally, people suffer severe traumatic amputations which they can survive. These amputations are avulsion in type and hence the limbs are unsuitable for reimplantation.

Injuries caused by penetrating missiles

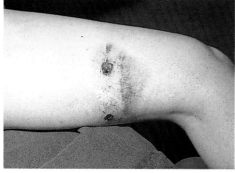
Simple gunshot wound showing entry and exit.

Free missiles travelling at speeds such that penetration of the body results are usually initiated by an explosive device. They include fragments from the casing of bombs, fragments from structures near the device, buckshot from a shotgun, and bullets from small firearms. Except for the case of bullets multiple injury is the rule, but similar pathology is caused by all missiles, and the subsequent management is common to all of the injuries.

Blast and gunshot injuries

These injuries are the most common after those caused by bomb explosions.

Injury is produced in two ways. Firstly, the missile may crush and lacerate tissue in its track, and if the anatomical configuration of the track passes through viscera or major blood vessels death or life threatening conditions may result. Secondly, during retardation of the missile some or all of its kinetic energy is transferred to the target; these wounds are classified according to whether or not the amount of energy transferred is such as to produce significant damage outside the track. Any of the missiles described may have the potential to produce a high energy transfer wound. Even if the exact circumstances are known it may be impossible to predict the degree of energy transfer. The amount of energy deposited for any given bullet will depend on its position in flight, the range, the weapon, and the type of target struck. In general, bullets from rifles and machine guns have a greater potential to produce high energy wounds than those from hand guns and most bomb fragments.

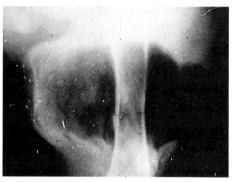

Radiograph showing cavitation effect within the tissues produced by high energy transfer.

The pathology produced by high energy transfer is tissue damage outside the missile track. Macroscopically there may be disruption of solid or semi-solid viscera, while in elastic tissues in the limbs there will be a stripping open of tissue planes for some distance from the track. Within the abdomen there may be disruption of hollow viscera caused by the associated pressure changes. Microscopically there will be large areas of non-homogeneous tissue damage with some cell death and much microvascular instability, producing ischaemia in some parts, which may be reversible. Such tissues are particularly prone to infection, especially by anaerobic bacteria.

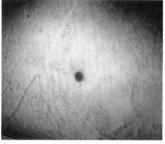
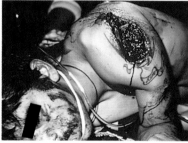

Shoulder wound caused by bomb fragment. Energy deposit damage and contamination (right) was found on exploration of what seemed to be a simple wound (left).

In nearly all missile wounds there will be contamination of the wound by foreign material, usually clothing. When low energy transfer occurs the material is usually carried into the wound on the front of the missile and remains close to it. In high energy transfer wounds foreign material is literally sucked into the wound through both entry and exit wounds, disrupted into minute fragments, and then distributed along dissected tissue planes, sometimes as far as 20-30 cm from the track. Clothing material is invariably highly contaminated with organisms. If the gastrointestinal tract is breached the bowel contents are distributed into all parts of the peritoneal cavity and along the extra-abdominal track.

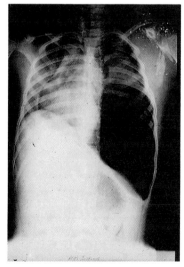

Gunshot wound of left shoulder with secondary tension pneumothorax.

Surgical exploration of high energy missile wounds is usually mandatory to remove dead tissue and foreign material and to provide ideal circumstances for the microcirculation to recover as rapidly as possible by ensuring that no tension develops in the wound. This may entail wide fasciotomy, leaving wounds open for delayed primary closure and preventing unnecessary movement, especially from unstable fractures. Although not a substitute for surgery, antibiotics may have an important role in helping to prevent infection, but these are effective only if given early.

The radiograph depicting blast lung is reproduced by kind permission of Mr R W Peyton and that of a gunshot wound to the shoulder by Mr J R Gibbons. The photograph depicting traumatic amputation and a shoulder wound caused by a bomb fragment and the radiograph showing cavitation have Crown copyright and are reproduced with the author's permission.

TRANSPORT OF INJURED PATIENTS

Alastair Wilson, Peter Driscoll

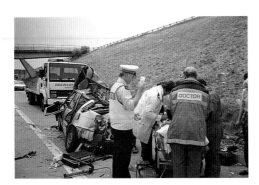

Victims of trauma begin dying immediately after their injuries have occurred. Prehospital care must provide early and expert resuscitation and then transportation to the most appropriate hospital for the patient's needs. This care begins with first aid administered by bystanders and ends with the fully coordinated response of the hospital's trauma team.

The criteria in the box are rarely met, and so the medical immediate care responder will have to make do with the facilities available in the locality.

Requirements for provision of effective prehospital care

- Public education in first aid and resuscitation
- An immediate communication system linking those at the accident site with ambulance control
- An instant computerised printout at ambulance control of the site from which the call has been made and the map reference
- Computerised identification of the nearest ambulance vehicles with grading of their medical expertise. (These vehicles require a computer printout of the accident location before being given full medical details)
- An intelligent sequence of questions and answers between the controller and the person reporting the accident
- Immediately available medical advice to the controller
- Excellent lines of communication with emergency vehicles and immediate care staff
- Adequate numbers of emergency vehicles with properly trained paramedics on board
- Uniform back up from doctors who can give immediate care
- Sensible triage with direct communication with the selected hospital
- Medical helicopter transport from distant or inaccessible sites to a network of hospitals and trauma units

---

Remember that accident sites are dangerous. Safety to self comes first. Ensure that you are immunised against tetanus and hepatitis. Wear appropriate clothing with reflective bands and designation labels, a helmet, and protective footwear. Watch for jagged metal edges, petrol and chemical spillages, and drivers who decide to get round the accident by driving on the hard shoulder. The patient should be moved instantly only if there is no chance of survival otherwise.

If you are not skilled in immediate care do not get in the way of those who are. Doctors inevitably have skills beyond those of the general public and should use them wisely and not panic.

It is a widely held belief that mortality in both the first and second half hours after injury increases by a factor of three if medical intervention is delayed. It is essential that delays are minimised and skilled medical intervention occurs as soon after injury as possible. Expert resuscitation must be given continuously during transport from the scene of the accident to the receiving hospital. Movement should not interrupt this process.

Resuscitation and immediate assessment

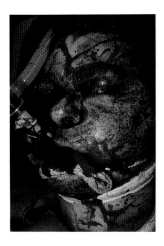

A rigid collar is used to protect the cervical spine of an accident victim.

There is no difference in principle between resuscitation in the accident and emergency department and that at the accident site, but greater impediments to a successful outcome face the first responder. Nevertheless he or she must keep a level head and work out the most efficient method of achieving the same end points as are achieved in the ordered surroundings of the hospital resuscitation room.

Airway

In assessing and maintaining the airway take into account the patient's level of consciousness and position, vomiting, facial fractures, entrapment, and environment. If the patient is unable to maintain an airway then secure it immediately, but remember that any injury above the clavicles indicates that a cervical spine injury may coexist. Protect the cervical spine, preferably with a rigid collar, simultaneously with airway assessment.

Transport of injured patients

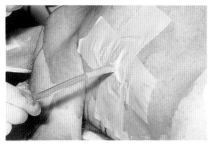

Chest drain in place.

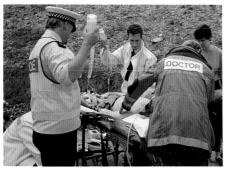

Crash victim with two intravenous lines in place.

Breathing

Monitoring the respiratory rate is an excellent method of determining the presence of respiratory difficulties. Rates greater than 30 breaths per minute and less than 15 per minute are abnormal. If breathing is compromised despite a patent airway assess and note the reason for the compromise. Patients with a pneumothorax or haemothorax must receive chest drainage if positive pressure ventilation is to be instituted. A flail chest or eventration of the diaphragm may demand positive pressure ventilation. Patients with severe head injuries become hypercapnic as their breathing deteriorates. Hypercapnia dilates vessels in the brain, exacerbating cerebral oedema and increasing intracranial pressure. This also demands ventilatory support.

Circulation

Replace lost blood with an adequate volume given through two large bore cannulas (14G or 16G). Remember to measure the blood pressure and heart rate. If bleeding is visible and controllable stem it by applying external pressure. It is helpful if a blood sample can be taken and sent for cross matching at the same time as the intravenous cannulas are inserted.

Dysfunction

Determine the patient's Glasgow coma scale score and pupillary response and check for spinal cord injuries by asking the patient to wiggle his or her fingers and toes. This does not totally rule out spinal cord injury, so if time allows determine the level of any sensory or motor defect.

Exposure

Exposure may cause hypothermia in the injured patient. If clothing is removed to facilitate access ensure that the patient is adequately covered and kept warm and dry.

Thoughout initial resuscitation the patient and the accident scene must be assessed and the mechanism of injury determined. Polaroid photography at the scene is of value.

Make an accurate record of all procedures performed and note the patient's responses. Injuries are recorded in anatomical order and physiological measurements summated as the triage revised trauma score. Prehospital care charts can act as an aide memoir.

The patient's condition determines the timing and type of transport that must be employed. He or she may require stabilisation at the accident site before transportation by road ambulance to a local hospital. Alternatively, specialist care at a more distant hospital may be required and transfer by helicopter should be considered. It may be impossible to stabilise the patient on site without complex intervention. If there is an appropriate hospital close by then the fastest possible transport with continuous resuscitation is indicated.

When a patient is taken to a non-specialist hospital there is often a delay of several hours before further transfer to a multidisciplinary or specialist unit can be arranged. It pays to get the patient to the right hospital in a single movement from the accident site.

Indications for direct transportation to a trauma unit have been laid down by Champion.[1] A slightly modified version of this list is given in the box. It is used to raise clinical suspicion of multisystem injury and the requirement for treatment in a multidisciplinary hospital.

Indications for direct transportation

- Penetrating injury to the chest, abdomen, head, neck, or groin
- Two or more proximal long bone fractures
- Burns covering >15% of body area or burns to the face or airway
- Evidence of high energy impactment
  - Falls of ≥6 m (≥20 ft)
  - Crash speed of ≥32 km/h (≥20 mph)
  - Inward deformity of the car of 0·6 m (2 ft)
  - Rearward displacement of the front axle
  - Intrusion of the passenger compartment of 38 cm (15 in) on the patient's side or 50 cm (20 in) on opposite side
  - Ejection of the patient
  - Rollover
  - Death of a car occupant
  - Pedestrian hit at ≥32 km/h (≥20 mph)
  - Abnormal values for physiological variables

Problems at the scene of accident

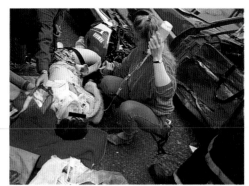

Patient trapped by his legs after a motorcycle accident.

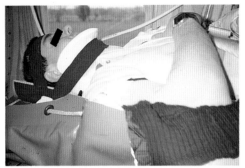

Russel Extraction Device and rigid cervical collar.

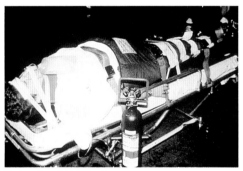

Patient in a MAST suit.

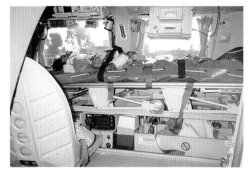

Interior of the London Crusader helicopter.

Entrapment

Victims of road traffic accidents are frequently trapped, and this complicates the management of serious injuries. The fire and rescue service is required to extricate all trapped people. Ensure that the service is summoned and maintain close coordination between medical, ambulance, and fire personnel. Throughout extrication the patient should receive the usual attention to the airway, breathing, and circulation. When compressed limbs are suddenly freed precipitate hypovolaemic shock may ensue. Maintain the blood pressure by giving intravenous fluids throughout extrication.

Once the patient has been freed from the wreckage assessment should continue. Note and correct detrimental changes to the airway, breathing, or circulation. The airway is of cardinal importance and must be secure before extrication. If an endotracheal tube is in place it is wise to disconnect it for the moment of extrication to avoid having to replace it. Although intravenous lines may be placed with less difficulty after extrication, their establishment must not be delayed, especially if extrication is likely to be prolonged, in patients with hypovolaemic shock or crushed limbs. External blood loss at any new site should be stopped by direct pressure.

If the patient is unconscious or the mechanism of the injury indicates that there may be spinal cord damage the neck must be stabilised before movement. Philadelphia or Stifneck collars, though ideal in the recumbent position, do not allow the patient's torso, neck, and head to be kept in constant relation to each other. For this purpose a Kendrick Extraction Device (KED) or Russell Extraction Device (RED) (spine immobilisers) should be used. Sometimes it is possible to slide a Vacumat extraction mattress under the patient to prevent unnecessary movement during extrication.

Analgesia

Adequate analgesia is important, especially in trapped patients. Entonox is of help only initially because over a period of time its intermittent analgesic effect is inadequate. Give subanaesthetic doses of opiates or ketamine as repeated intravenous boluses. If opiates are used give an antiemetic and monitor blood pressure and level of consciousness.

Packaging and stabilising the patient before transportation

The principle that underpins successful movement and transportation is that of preventing further injury. All forms of transport entail movement that subjects the injured patient to energy changes that are inherently harmful. Excessive abnormal movement of broken limbs may compromise vessels; moving the head on the torso can dislocate a precarious cervical spine. Maximum energy changes occur as stretchers are manhandled into vehicles. A swollen brain becomes more swollen the more it is moved within the cranium, and if an unrestrained patient moves about in the back of an ambulance as it brakes, accelerates, and turns corners further damage is inevitable. Each movement imparts further injury, so avoid unnecessary movement.

Patients' conditions deteriorate during transportation. Airways and intravenous lines may become disconnected or be removed. Anticipate the worst possible occurrences before moving. Check that the most appropriate airway is being used. If the patient is breathing spontaneously but has a reduced level of consciousness ensure that a sucker is at hand and that a Trendelenberg tilt can be obtained on the stretcher. A nasogastric tube ensures an empty stomach.

Most patients are transported supine because spinal injuries cannot be excluded. Managing the patient in a lateral position is inappropriate if a cervical injury has not been excluded but otherwise is much safer. If a pneumothorax or haemothorax is present treat it immediately by using a large bore chest drain (32-36 FG) in the axilla, connected through a Portex chest drainage bag.

The airway is best protected with a cuffed endotracheal tube, but remember that the neck may be unstable and a nasal tube or cricothyrotomy may be more appropriate. Check that the tube is absolutely secure and in the right place. If a ventilator is being used a disconnect alarm in the circuit is helpful. Portable pulse oximeters and end tidal carbon dioxide detectors are useful for the early detection of ventilatory mishap.

Transport of injured patients

Before transportation check that:

- The airway is clear and secured
- Breathing is symmetrical and not compromised
- Two intravenous lines are in place and accessible
- The spine is properly mobilised
- All monitoring equipment is working
- Drugs and equipment are at hand

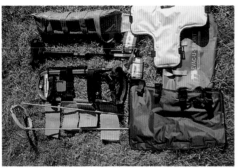

A variety of limb splints.

Insert intravenous lines away from joints, but if they are inserted in the antecubital fossa a purpose designed Armback is helpful in keeping the arm straight and securing the lines. A confused patient must be adequately restrained or, if this is impossible, paralysed. Ensure that the whole spine is protected. Remember that dislocations occur at spinal levels other than in the cervical region. Care of the spine extends throughout the length of the vertebral column.

The patient who either has hypovolaemic shock or is likely to develop it requires intravenous infusion. Check that large bore cannulas have been inserted peripherally and are working. There are few indications for central line insertion at the scene of an accident, and the practice may be harmful. If possible blood should be taken when the intravenous lines are inserted and sent on for cross matching at the receiving hospital.

Limb splintage

The aim of splintage is to prevent further damage to soft tissue and the compromise of the vascular supply of a limb. The appropriate splint must be chosen. Compressing pneumatic splints or MAST anti-shock trousers are useful for reducing blood loss from pelvic and leg fractures. If blood loss is not a problem non-compromising traction splints allow easier inspection of the limb and palpation of pulses. It may help to place the patient on a conforming mattress such as the Evacumat, which can be curved about his or her limbs, torso, head, and neck. These are only semirigid.

Timing

Speed is of the essence. The time taken to stabilise the airway and institute effective ventilation, control of bleeding, and limb and spinal splintage and to initiate volume replacement should never exceed 15 minutes, and the target time for completing these tasks is 10 minutes.

Transportation

Essential information to be given to the receiving hospital

- Age and sex of the patient
- Mechanism of injury
- Vital signs at the scene
- Initial findings on assessment
- Procedures performed at the scene
- Response to procedures
- Estimated time of arrival

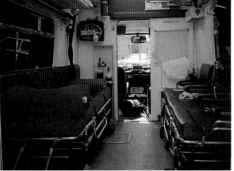

Interior of a typical land ambulance.

The transport phase is often regarded as a therapeutic vacuum in which no treatment is possible. The speed of an ambulance flashing a blue light in London is only 6 km/h faster than its routine speed. The use of the two tone siren is effective in terrifying the passing motorist but also terrifies the patient.

During transport more practical procedures can be carried out. Further intravenous lines may be set up and small fractures can be splinted. A more thorough assessment of the patient's condition is possible, and monitoring and recording of the vital signs must be continued throughout.

Staff in the receiving hospital must be informed of the patient's impending arrival and condition by the ambulance staff, and in the light of the information, staff in the emergency department must prepare the resuscitation room and summon the trauma team (this is discussed in the article on initial assessment).

Potential problems

(1) The sudden development of respiratory distress may require precipitate ventilation. Make sure that the patient is positioned with his or her head next to the attendant's seat and that there is room to gain access to the airway and that the visibility is adequate for placing an endotracheal tube.
(2) The development of a tension pneumothorax in a ventilated patient necessitates insertion of a large bore cannula (14 G) in the second intercostal space in the midclavicular line.
(3) Unexpected cardiac arrest requires cardiopulmonary resuscitation. The presence of two attendants ensures complete control of the patient and prevents ineffective therapeutic measures that would result from a single operator.

Land ambulance

Some ambulances have facilities to monitor blood pressure, heart rate, and cardiac rhythm. It is not wise to rely on an electrocardiogram as artefacts caused by movement interfere with the tracing, and even a good trace does not reflect adequate tissue perfusion. Pulse oximetry is useful but has limitations because a reasonable cardiac output is a prerequisite. Adequate lighting and space are essential.

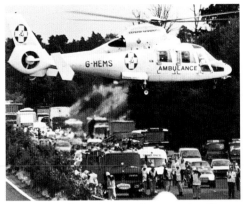

The London Crusader attending a road traffic accident.

Helicopter transport

Indications
- Requirements for specialist trauma centre care
- Long distances
- Obstruction to land transport by traffic.
- Obscure or inaccessible accident site
- Need for interhospital transfer of critically ill patients
- Need for transportation of medical staff or equipment to the accident scene

Contraindications
- Weather conditions
- Difficulty with landing helicopters because of local obstructions or poor lighting
- The patient's injuries are not sufficient to warrant specialised care in specialised units
- Patients who are violent or have psychiatric problems
- The incident has occurred close to the most appropriate hospital for the patient's needs

Handing over the patient

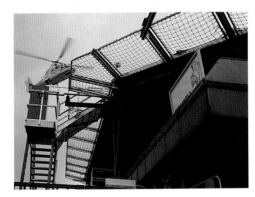

The air ambulance landing on the helipad on the roof of The Royal London Hospital.

Air ambulance

The designated medical helicopter is the most expensive part of the prehospital medical armamentarium and should be used with care. In particular it should carry crew who are trained to the highest possible level and who will act as the extended arm of the hospital. Because the helicopter can be used for long and short transportations as well as for secondary transport from primary hospitals to tertiary multidisciplinary centres it requires full monitoring facilities, which include:

- A non-invasive blood pressure monitor
- A defibrillator
- An electrocardiograph and pulse rate monitor
- Invasive blood pressure monitors
- Temperature monitors
- Syringe drivers and infusions pumps
- Suckers
- Ventilators
- A pulse oximeter and pulse rate monitor
- A capnograph

There are problems concerned with the use of helicopters that are not specifically designed for medical transportation (for example, police craft) in that they are not permitted to carry cardiac monitors, non-invasive blood pressure monitors, and oximeters as they can emit electromagnetic radiation, which interferes with the helicopter's avionics. Furthermore, they are cramped, with minimal equipment, and may be dangerous once in the air because there is such a limited capacity for responding to any emergency. Anticipating potential problems is even more important than during land transport. Anticipate problems before lift off or ensure that the necessary equipment and space to cope with them are available during flight.

Helicopters are noisy, and interpersonal communications can be difficult. Headphones should be placed on the patient's head to allow reassuring conversation. (Do not play soothing music.) The patient should be kept warm and comfortable during the transport. If a long journey is expected an antiemetic may be given to prevent air sickness, and the stomach should be kept empty by frequent gastric aspiration.

The helicopter should be summoned early by contacting the appropriate ambulance headquarters. Ideally, the police, the fire brigade, and land ambulance staff should have access to the telephone number.

All details about the accident and any changes in the patient's condition during transport must be communicated to the emergency department staff. This takes time. Although the information categories are as before, it is important that ambulance staff or first responders do not suddenly disappear while the resuscitation team are attending to their protocols. This means that the team delivering the patient must remain with the patient until the trauma team leader is certain that he or she has noted all of the relevant details. It is often wise to wait a little longer, because afterthoughts are routine. It is particularly important that the patient's response to procedures that have occurred during transportation are communicated to the emergency staff and improvements or deteriorations in physiological scores in the presence of varying degrees of resuscitation efforts are noted.

1 Jones I, Champion H. Trauma triage: vehicle damage as an estimate of injury severity. *J Trauma* 1989;**29**:646-53.

We thank Dr C Carney, Dr J Lloyd-Parry, Mr P Birchinall, and Mr A Newton for helpful comments.

Recommended standards for medical helicopter systems

A working party has made recommendations for minimum acceptable standards of safety for patients, staff, and the community regarding definitions of primary and secondary medical flights; organisation, acceptance of transfers, and conduct of care; definition and responsibilities of the medical director; doctors; nurses and paramedical staff; pilots; staffing procedures; training; installation and minimal levels of equipment; neonatal transfers; protocols; audit and record keeping; major disasters; and confidentiality. Copies of the recommendations can be obtained from the chairman, Dr Aubrey Bristow, consultant anaesthetist, St Bartholomew's Hospital, London.

MAJOR ACCIDENTS

Stephen Miles

Major accidents affect individual hospitals rarely, but when they occur they cause total disruption of the hospital's normal activities. Large numbers of casualties arrive within a short space of time, and the presence of police and media representatives may complicate the proceedings considerably. To avoid chaos developing on such occasions the full implications of a major accident need to be considered, full major accident plans should be prepared, and adequate staff training must be undertaken.

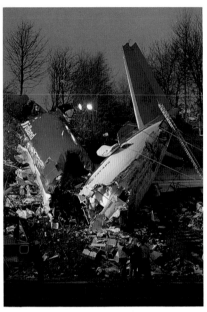

M1 aeroplane crash at Kegworth.

Clapham rail disaster.

Types of major accident

- Large fires — Bradford stadium, King's Cross
- Explosions—chemical — Flixborough
  - —gas — Putney
  - —bombs — Old Bailey, Hyde Park
- Public transport disasters—air — Tenerife, M1 (Kegworth)
  - —rail — Moorgate, Clapham
  - —road — M4 coach crash, multiple pile ups
  - —sea — Zeebrugge
- Buildings collapsing — Ronan point
- Nuclear disasters — Chernobyl, Three Mile Island
- Riots — Wapping, Tottenham

Major accidents will cause a variable number of deaths, depending on the nature and severity of the event, but among the survivors the pattern is similar in virtually all cases—that is, there is a relatively small number of patients requiring immediate or urgent treatment and a large number of patients with minor injuries.

The actual number of patients the hospital is prepared to cope with should not be left to chance; a careful review of resources should establish how many patients in each category the hospital is able to deal with, and this figure should be communicated to the emergency services for incorporation into their own major accident plans. Each hospital will thus receive only a finite number of casualties, any additional patients being taken to other hospitals in the area.

Factors in major accident planning

- Staff resources
  - —medical
  - —nursing
  - —administrative
- Hospital resources
  - —space in accident and emergency department
  - —number of intensive care unit beds
  - —number of theatres
  - —equipment
- Special factors in area
  - —nuclear plants
  - —chemical plants
  - —inner city area (bombs, riots)
  - —motorways
  - —airports
- Availability of support from nearby hospitals

When dealing with victims of a major accident most hospital staff are called on to perform in exactly the same way as they do at other times, albeit under considerable pressure. A small number of staff have specialised duties, which are described below.

Initiation of major accident procedure

Designated hospital

- First informed
- Receives details of accident, estimated number of casualties, etc
- Provides site medical officer and (if required) mobile medical teams
- Receives first wave of casualties

Supporting hospitals

- Receive casualties when designated hospital is not able to cope
- If close to scene of accident may provide site medical officer and mobile teams so that designated hospital retains valuable staff

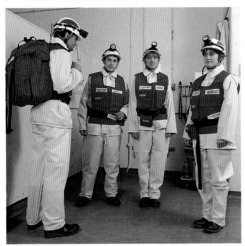

Emergency medical team in protective clothing.

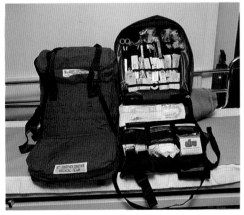

Equipment carried by medical team.

As far as the hospital is concerned a major accident is any event that results in live casualties of a number and with injuries of a severity that call for extraordinary measures to be taken for their reception and treatment. The emergency services sometimes view things from their own perspective and may take refuge in a figure of 50 casualties as a trigger point for declaring a major accident. This is unhelpful to hospitals as 10 patients with serious injuries are far more difficult to cope with than 70 patients with minor injuries. Senior hospital staff may therefore sometimes have to take the decision to initiate the major accident procedure themselves.

Notification of major accidents, however, generally comes from the emergency services, usually the ambulance service, and comes to the hospital switchboard or the accident and emergency department. Information is given about the nature of the accident, the number of live casualties expected, and whether the hospital is a *designated* or *supporting* hospital. A designated hospital will receive the bulk of the casualties and will be the first to receive them. A supporting hospital will receive the overflow that the designated hospital is unable to deal with.

The notification of a major accident is often staged: as the declaration of a major accident causes considerable disruption and expense the emergency services understandably want to be sure that it is justified. Therefore such a declaration can be made only by a senior officer, and, while he or she is on the way to the scene, emergency vehicles that have already arrived report by radio to their headquarters.

When it is clear that something serious has occurred the designated hospital generally receives a *major accident warning*. Some hospitals do not take any specific action on receiving such a warning, but this is unwise. If the accident has occurred close to the hospital patients may begin to arrive within a few minutes, and a major accident may never be formally declared, either owing to confusion at the scene or because the senior officer present does not consider the declaration justified from his or her service's point of view.

For the reasons mentioned above when a major accident warning is received immediate preparatory action should begin. The medical, nursing, and administrative coordinators (described below) should assemble and establish a *control centre*. They should initiate the administrative measures required by the major accident procedure and summon the site medical officer and members of emergency medical teams to the control centre so that their presence may be noted. These personnel can then begin changing into protective clothing and assembling their equipment. It is appropriate to dispatch the site medical officer to the scene at this point.

The patients already in the accident and emergency department also have to be considered, and measures must be taken to empty the department. If the major accident warning turns out to have been a false alarm valuable practice in initiating the major accident procedure will have been gained by all participants; if the incident develops the hospital will be well on the way to being prepared for the reception of casualties.

Site organisation

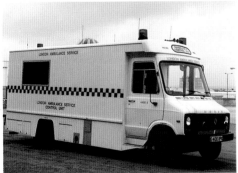

Emergency ambulance control vehicle.

On hearing of a major accident the emergency services always dispatch special emergency control vehicles to the scene. These are equipped with sophisticated communication systems and control the activities of members of their services who are working at the scene. The fire service is mainly concerned with evacuating casualties as well as controlling fire, smoke, and other hazards. The ambulance service is also concerned in evacuating casualties, administering first aid to them, and transporting them to hospital. The police are in charge overall at the scene and are responsible for sealing off the area, clearing roads to the hospital, keeping away unwanted sightseers, and identifying casualties. The three services each have a designated incident officer, and these liaise with each other. Hospital personnel arriving at the scene make contact with the ambulance control vehicle and the attending ambulance incident officer.

Major accidents

Duties of the site medical officer

- Liaise with emergency services
- Assess the scene
- Report to base hospital number of casualties and severity of injuries
- Inform emergency services if hospital unable to cope
- Check that mobile medical teams have the equipment they require
- Watch teams for signs of fatigue and arrange for replacements
- Notify hospital when the last casualty has left the scene

The site medical officer does not participate in treating patients

Clothing for site medical officer and mobile medical teams

- Safety helmet with headlight
- Bright reflective and waterproof clothing
- Tabards with designation clearly displayed ("doctor," "nurse")
- Wellington boots or other robust footwear

Equipment to be carried to scene of accident

Intravenous giving sets and cannulas
Plastic bottles of colloid solution
Sphygmomanometer, tourniquets
Intubation equipment
Stethoscopes
Suction equipment
Face masks and Guedel airways
Ambu bag
Chest drainage kit
Suturing kit with suture materials
Amputation kit
Drug box containing morphine, tranquillisers, anaesthetic drugs (for amputation)
Syringes and needles
Inflatable splints
Scissors and pens
Bandages and dressings (various)
Adhesive strapping
Triage labels

Triage categories

Category	Example
(1) Immediate	Head injury with unequal pupils and developing neurological signs
(2) Urgent	Suspected ruptured spleen or pneumothorax
(3) Minor	Cuts, bruises, and minor fractures
(4) Palliative	60 Year old patient with 80% burns
(5) Dead	

Site medical officer/medical incident officer

The site medical officer is often, and with some logic, known as the medical incident officer and is generally the first doctor on the scene. He or she represents the hospital and liaises with the ambulance incident officer. It is important that the site medical officer does not attend to patients as this would compromise his or her other duties.

The question of who should fill the role of site medical officer is a vexed one. Traditionally it has been allocated to physicians, as they are not required at the hospital to treat casualties and, lacking surgical expertise, are less likely to concern themselves with treating patients at the scene. Unfortunately these doctors are likely to be completely at sea when confronted with the horrors of a major accident and may lack the authority to deal effectively with the emergency services.

The members of the British Association for Immediate Care (BASICS) specialise in rescue work and regularly participate in practice exercises. If there is a BASICS organisation close to the hospital it may be appropriate to enlist its services.

Mobile medical teams

The hospital may also be requested to provide mobile medical teams, normally consisting of a surgeon, an anaesthetist, and two to four nurses. They should be appropriately dressed and carry equipment in backpacks.

Heavy suitcases and boxes full of equipment are of little value in the awkward situations that may confront the teams at the scene of a major accident, and their transport to the scene from the nearest access point requires deployment of personnel that could better be used in evacuating and caring for casualties. The equipment to be carried is a matter of local choice, but the list in the box gives an idea of the range of items that should be carried. These should be divided appropriately among the various members of the team so that, for example, the anaesthetist has all the equipment required for care of the airway and the nurses have a reasonable supply of dressings. It is not usually necessary to carry oxygen in the packs as most ambulances have cylinders of it on board.

Apart from providing first aid and necessary treatment for patients with serious injuries the principal task of the site medical teams is to assess the patients as rapidly as possible and divide them into triage categories. This will enable the most severely injured patients to be transported to hospital first. This should be obvious; but, unfortunately, unless this procedure is carefully executed, the patients most likely to be transported first are the ones making the most noise, and these are frequently the least severely injured.

Once the patients have been allocated to triage categories, they should be labelled accordingly with clear reflective labels. Suitable labels are available from BASICS, and these have the advantage that the triage category of the patient may readily be altered if his or her condition warrants it. Such labelling at the scene of the accident not only helps in the orderly evacuation of the casualties but also makes for smoother reception of patients at the hospital.

Some patients may be trapped and may require drips, pain relief, etc, until they can be freed. Very occasionally it proves impossible, even with heavy cutting gear, to release a trapped person, and in these rare cases limb amputation may have to be considered.

Hospital organisation

The key to the successful running of a major accident procedure lies in establishing an *effective control centre*. This should be staffed by medical, nursing, and administrative coordinators, with appropriate support staff; all should be of the most senior rank possible (for example, an accident and emergency consultant, a senior nursing officer, a senior administrator) and be thoroughly familiar with the major accident procedure. They should liaise continuously to ensure that it is running smoothly.

Medical coordinator

Once the medical coordinator has established the control centre in conjunction with the two other coordinators his or her first priorities are to clear the accident and emergency department; to dispatch the site medical officer to the scene; and to organise the mobile medical teams, ensure that they are properly dressed and equipped, and arrange transport for them. Once this is done the chief task is to recruit and organise the medical staff. The medical coordinator has to check that the switchboard is calling in appropriate staff and summoning junior staff from residences and has to designate a relatively senior member of staff (usually a surgeon) to be *triage officer*. The triage officer receives the casualties at the ambulance entrance and allocates them to triage categories if this has not already been done at the scene; if it has been done he or she reassesses the patient's condition to ensure that the original designation is still correct and, having made this decision on triage, then allocates the patients to appropriate areas within the department.

The medical coordinator also has to organise medical staff as they arrive. This is an important task as staff commonly arrive in excessive numbers and may cause considerable confusion by acting independently without referring to the coordinator. At least two doctors are required for the resuscitation of any critically injured patients, and, if possible, one doctor should be allocated to each stretcher patient. A single doctor, supported by nurses, will be able to care for all of the patients with minor injuries until more medical staff become available.

Most staff working in the accident and emergency department during a major accident procedure will not be fully familiar with its functioning. Officials and regular accident and emergency staff should be clearly identified so that they may help in locating supplies of intravenous equipment, drugs, etc.

The medical coordinator also needs to establish, with the help of the nursing coordinator, which beds are available for those requiring admission and, in particular, what intensive care and theatre resources are required and how they may be provided. He or she should check that the doctors attending to the casualties are not becoming exhausted and ensure that they receive refreshments as required. Later on the medical coordinator may be required to address a press conference if requested by the hospital administration.

Nursing coordinator

The nursing coordinator's role is basically similar to that of the medical coordinator. He or she has to recruit nurses to go with the mobile medical teams and also to attend the patients in the accident and emergency department. Up to four nurses may be required for the resuscitation of a critically injured patient, and one nurse should be provided for each stretcher patient. In addition, the nursing coordinator should ensure that sufficient beds are cleared for the admission of patients with serious injuries and that patients who have been prematurely discharged to make way for the victims of the major accident are properly cared for.

Duties of the administrative coordinator

- Ensure that clerical staff are stationed to collect basic information about patients as they arrive (on specially designed stationery)
- Organise security and portering staff to direct relatives, public, and press away from treatment area and organise erection of signs
- Organise police control point and press area and equip them with telephones
- Designate other administrative staff to act as press officer, patient information officer, police liaison officer, etc
- Check switchboard is coping with overload of calls and that call out of off duty staff is proceeding smoothly
- Ensure catering, pharmacy, and supply needs are met

Stand down of the major accident procedure can occur when:

- Information has been received from the site that all casualties have been transported
- All affected departments in the hospital have been notified

Action cards for individual members of staff.

Administrative coordinator

The administrative coordinator has perhaps the most complex role, and it is one that needs to be practised. The successful running of a major accident procedure requires a great deal of documentation and record keeping: firstly, to keep track of patients, particularly if they are to be discharged; secondly, to provide the police with the identification information that they require for running their casualty bureau; and, finally, to answer inquiries from relatives who arrive at the hospital. The administrative incident officer has to set up a room for the police to operate in so that they can collate their information and perform any necessary interviews. He or she has to organise a proper press area in a place suitably remote from the accident and emergency department, and arrange to brief the press at regular intervals. Porters and security staff have to be organised to ensure that patients are transported expeditiously and that unwanted people are kept out of the treatment area. An area for relatives has to be established, together with a quiet room for interviews with the bereaved.

As the incident proceeds the administrative coordinator has to keep checking that the switchboard is coping with the avalanche of incoming calls it tends to receive on such occasions and that the operators have been able to contact all the necessary personnel. He or she also has to attend to medical supplies and catering needs.

This infrastructure is highly complicated but is absolutely essential if the doctors and nurses are to be able to treat the victims of the accident expeditiously.

When information is received from an official at the site that the last casualty has been taken from the scene and when all patients have either been admitted or discharged the three coordinators decide on a *stand down* of the major accident procedure.

After the stand down staff need to be debriefed. At the least this entails recording details of events that have occurred during the major accident procedure while their memories are still fresh. Staff may also require counselling if they are overexcited or upset, and temporal needs such as meals and transport home must be considered.

Major accident plan

A hospital cannot possibly organise itself to receive the victims of a major accident without detailed planning beforehand. This planning is incorporated into what is usually a weighty document known as the *Major Accident Plan*. This contains details of all the actions that everyone associated with the incident will have to take, from consultants to catering staff. It is unrealistic to expect individual members of staff to be familiar with the entire plan, so their portions of the plan should be summarised in individual documents known as *Action Cards*. These should be distributed to all members of staff likely to have to use them in the event of a major accident. No plan is perfect, and all potential participants need to be tested by some form of practice. This also serves the valuable purpose of staff training. Such exercises may be simply to test communications, when the switchboard operators attempt to contact all the staff they would have to if a major accident occurred; or they may be more elaborate affairs that employ mock casualties—these are difficult to run and have a tendency to degenerate into farce; the emergency services occasionally organise large scale major accident exercises, and hospitals in the vicinity should seek to participate in these.

The photograph of the M1 disaster was supplied by EMPICS, that of the Clapham disaster by Frank Spooner Pictures, and that of the emergency control vehicle by Mr C A J Keevil. Other photographs were taken by the education and medical illustration services department, St Bartholomew's Hospital.

Chemical accidents

Virginia Murray

Major chemical accidents cause problems for accident and emergency departments that are different from those recognised in other major accidents, for example, identification of toxin, the risk of cross chemical contamination of staff, and difficulties in patient management such as the need for ventilator equipment and antidotes. Therefore, particular attention should be given to preparation and planning.

What are the local chemical hazards?

Accident and emergency departments may find it useful to develop links with the area health and safety executive; local and county authorities, including the emergency planning officers; local emergency services such as the fire brigade; and local companies to identify factories or sites where hazardous substances may be stored or used. Many of these agencies will have information on assessment, control, and mitigation in the event of accidents, much of which concludes with "seek medical advice."

What accident and emergency department facilities are required?

Accident and emergency department facilities for decontamination and isolation should be identified; a study has shown many of these to be inadequate.[1] Major disaster equipment should include locally suitable protective clothing, and breathing apparatus if there are staff trained in its use. Frequent rehearsals with the equipment and facilities should be performed.

How can the poisons centres help?

The poisons centres are essential resources for managing the medical aspects of chemical accidents (see box). In certain situations they can notify and collaborate with other agencies concerned in investigation and epidemiological follow up and may also be able to provide on site toxicological advice and support. Their telephone numbers should be readily available.

Actions

When an incident occurs the accident and emergency department must obtain as much information as possible about the chemical(s) involved.

At the site—Protection of mobile medical team staff is essential, though there is no single set of protective clothing suitable for protection against every chemical. They should provide medical aid or triage only if told it is safe to do so, seek advice, and stay in communication with the emergency services control centres. Preferably only decontaminated casualties should be attended. (Decontamination facilities are provided only for fire brigade staff but are frequently used for casualties. However, these are usually suitable only for vertical patients and provide only cold water decontamination.) For the benefit of the casualty and the staff all contaminated clothing should be removed, bagged, and sealed, preferably at the site. Therefore, in addition to other medical equipment, consider taking surgical gowns or other clothing for casualties. Chemical contamination of skin and eyes may require prolonged irrigation or even immersion of affected part.

At the accident and emergency department—The above principles also apply to casualties arriving at hospital. Prior notification of an incident allows final preparation of hospital decontamination and isolation facilities by senior staff. Collection of blood, urine, vomit, and other relevant biological samples is valuable for confirming exposure and dose received and should be carried out as soon as possible after an incident.

1 Dallos V. Immediate response: accident and emergency departments. In: Murray V, ed. *Major chemical disasters: medical aspect of management.* London: Royal Society of Medicine, 1990:73-8. (International Congress and Symposium Series 155.)

HANDLING DISTRESSED RELATIVES AND BREAKING BAD NEWS

C A J McLauchlan

Problems associated with breaking bad news in cases of trauma

- Death or severe injury is sudden and unexpected
- The victim is often young
- The prognosis is often unsure
- Staff are often very busy
- Relatives may already have been notified in an unskilled manner
- The victim may have committed suicide
- Alcohol intoxication may have been a contributing factor

Coping with major trauma is stressful for both staff and the relatives. Handling distressed relatives is an underemphasised part of the work, and medical staff may have had no training and little experience of it. It is a time that the relative will always remember and, if handled badly, will leave lasting scars.

Various outcomes of major trauma

- Death
- Serious head injury
- Multiple injuries
- Spinal injury
- Major burns
- Loss of a limb
- Loss of sight

Giving bad news is never easy, but it can be especially difficult in cases of major trauma. The nature of the patient's problem and the bad news can be very varied. The management of the relatives may begin before they arrive at hospital and carry on until well after death or discharge of the patient. The principles of management apply to the accident and emergency department as well as the intensive treatment unit or admitting ward. Providing genuine understanding and support for relatives is the key to their management.

Initial contact

When a victim of major trauma arrives in the emergency room the priority is immediate resuscitation. Once the victim has been identified the closest relatives or friends should be notified.

Communication with the emergency services is very important. The ambulance crew and police, as well as giving information on the incident, may have already seen the relatives or know their whereabouts. It is usually better for a sympathetic police officer to make the initial contact in person rather than for a telephone call to be made from the hospital. The police may also be able to help with transport.

Handling the initial contact with relatives

- It may be preferable for a police officer to make contact in person
- Information on the telephone should be given by an experienced nurse or doctor
- Relatives should not drive to hospital alone
- The full severity of injuries or death may be best explained at the hospital

---

If the telephone is used information should be given by an experienced nurse or doctor and a lone relative advised strongly against driving to hospital alone. Mentioning that the victim is unconscious often helps to impart a certain severity to the lay person, although the full severity or death is usually best explained in person at the hospital. If relatives are not told of the victim's death, however, they may blame themselves for not arriving at the hospital in time to be with their loved one at death. It is important to dispel any self recrimination by giving the relatives the exact information, including the time of death. If the relatives have to travel great distances or from overseas the full details, including death, may have to be explained over the telephone. Find out if the relative is alone and, if so, suggest that he or she seeks support locally. Offer to telephone for support.

Arrival of relatives at the hospital

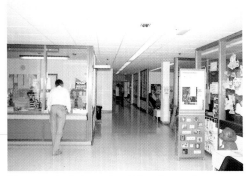

Distressed relatives should be given privacy and not kept waiting in reception areas, which may be impersonal and busy.

Anxious relatives should be met by a nurse and not be kept waiting around at reception for the department's or ward's communications to be established. Therefore, it is important that the nursing sister coordinates the information so that the staff, in particular those at reception, know that potentially distressed relatives are expected. They should be welcomed and not made to feel in the way. Staff should remember that it is not only the victim's relatives who may be distressed: in some instances close friends may be severely distressed and should be handled in the same way as the relatives.

There should be a private room or office where relatives and friends can wait and be seen. Ideally this room should be solely for relatives and friends and be suitably furnished.

Breaking the news

Essential features of a relatives' room

- Privacy
- Telephone
- Hand basin
- Mirror
- Appropriate decor and furniture
- Advice and information leaflets (out of sight)
- Tea cups

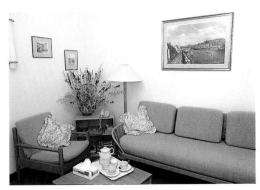

Relatives' room.

Remember to ask relatives for the medical history of the patient. This history may be vital if the patient is receiving certain drugs such as steroids or anticoagulants, and an idea of the quality of life may be useful in elderly victims or those with disease. Providing a history can also make relatives feel less helpless and that they are doing something.

During attempted resuscitation relatives should at least be given early warning if the condition is critical. Regular updates by the same person (usually a nurse) are also appreciated and may help to break the bad news in stages. It also allows relationships to form, which will help in providing the support that may be needed later.

The contact nurse should introduce a doctor, preferably a senior one to the relatives as soon as possible to provide further information. Relatives expect to see a doctor for medical information and an idea of the prognosis: "Will he be alright, doctor?"

Advice for the doctor

Breaking bad news has to be tailored to the situation and the particular relatives, but the following principles generally apply:

- On leaving the resuscitation area or theatre you may be stressed, so take a moment to compose yourself and think about what you are going to say. Also remove evidence of blood stains, etc, so that you are physically and mentally prepared

- Take an experienced nurse with you. A nurse can be a great support and can carry on where you leave off

- Confirm that you have the correct relatives and who's who. Ascertain what information they already have

- Enter the relatives' room, introduce yourself, and sit down near the patient's closest relative. Do not stand holding the door handle like a bus conductor ready to jump out. Giving the impression that you have time to talk and listen is important

- In general look at who your are talking to, be honest and direct, and keep it simple. Be prepared to emphasise the main points. Avoid too much technical information at this stage (although with patients with multiple injuries there may be much going on). If death is probable say so; do not beat about the bush

- After breaking bad news allow time and some moments of silence while the facts sink in

- Be prepared for a variety of emotional responses or reactions. Some people may stick at one reaction whereas others go through several reactions

- Allow and encourage reactions such as crying. Provide tissues and facilities for relatives to make themselves presentable to the world again

- Although it is upsetting, close relatives appreciate the truth and your honest empathy

- At this stage there is no substitute for genuine understanding and support. A sensitive nurse is a great asset

Some immediate grief reactions

- Numbness—that is, acceptance but no feeling
- Disbelief
- Acute distress
- Anger—including that against the medical care; blaming themselves or others
- Guilt
- Acceptence

Handling distressed relatives and breaking bad news

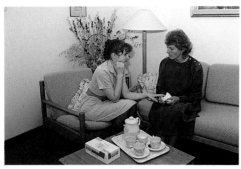

A sensitive nurse is a great asset after the news has been broken.

• Tea usually appears, and this is another sign that the relatives' distress is appreciated

• During the interview it is a helpful and natural comfort for staff to touch or hold the hand of the relative. Various social and cultural factors may influence the appropriateness of touching, but generally if it comes naturally then it is probably right

• Likewise, during the interview it may be natural for the staff to have sad feelings, and these need not be completely hidden. Some sign of emotion may help distressed or bereaved people to realise that the staff do have some understanding and it is not just another case

• Avoid platitudes—for example, after a death comments such as "you've still got your other son, etc," which are not helpful as it is the dead person whom the relatives want back. Also avoid false sympathy as in "I know what it's like," but rather empathise, as in: "It must be hard for you. . ." or "It must feel very unreal. . .," etc, reflecting back their emotions.

Encourage and be prepared for questions to be asked during the interview. These may disclose any misunderstandings and present a chance to re-emphasise the message. The question of pain and suffering is common and should be discussed routinely, with reassurance as appropriate. The prognosis may be unknown initially, and you should say so. If death or serious disability is possible, however, then it is only fair to be honest and warn the relatives. It will be a worse shock later if they have been protected from this knowledge. Do not be afraid to answer that you do not know the answers to medical or philosophical questions such as "Why me?" Other difficult questions may arise from feelings of guilt or when a relative was involved in but not injured in the same accident. Special problems may arise if the relative feels responsible directly—for example, as the driver in an accident. Other complications may include a recent squabble before the accident with subsequent self recrimination. The "If only. . ." rumination can be a type of guilt response that is fruitless and should be understood but discouraged at the outset.

If death has already occurred the same principles as discussed above apply. It is important to use the word "death" or "dead" early and avoid euphemisms such as "passed on." The news is usually hard to accept and so it must be as clear as possible, abrupt as it may seem. People usually need an explanation as to the cause of death of a loved one. It may be helpful to explain the inevitability in the light of known injuries and that "everything possible was done." Worries about their own first aid at the scene of the accident may need talking through.

Children should not be excluded from the proceedings in the mistaken belief that they need protection. They will be afraid and may have fantasies and feelings of guilt and need information.

Staff actions during the interview with the bereaved

Allow
• Time
• The bereaved to react
• Silence
• Touching
• Questions

Avoid
• Rushing
• "Protecting" from the truth
• Platitudes
• False sympathy
• Euphemisms

Whenever possible relatives should be given a clear explanation of the cause of death

---

Management of relatives

Reality is preferable to fantasy so allow relatives to see even critically ill patients, albeit briefly

Seeing the patient

Depending on urgency of further treatment it should usually be possible for close relatives briefly to see the patient before he or she is rushed off to theatre, the intensive treatment unit, or even another hospital. Although distressing, reality is usually preferable to fantasy. Also, sometimes this may be the last time that they will see their loved one alive. In addition, this contact may be beneficial to the conscious patient. Relatives may ask to enter or remain in the resuscitation area during emergency treatment, especially of infants and children. This is not yet generally accepted, but it seems that it can be beneficial provided that they are supported by an advocate such as a sensitive member of staff (for example, a relative who is a witness may better appreciate both the seriousness of the situation and the vigour of resuscitation efforts). Hospital staff may, however, be apprehensive about the presence of relatives, and their feelings must be considered.

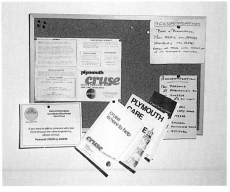

Useful information in the relatives' room.

Seeing the body after death

The opportunity to see the body after death should always be offered and gently encouraged if there is any doubt. Well meaning friends may try and discourage this act, which is an important part of accepting reality.

The imagination is usually far worse than reality, and cruel fantasies about the victim being disfigured or squashed flat can be dispelled. The actions and words of staff when relatives are with the body should give "permission" for relatives to touch, hold, kiss, or say goodbye to their loved one. Nurses will often carefully prepare a body before viewing in the clinical area or chapel. The relative may also like to be left alone with the body.

Checklist of actions in the event of death

- Notify the general practitioner, other relatives and friends, and the coroner's officer

- Ensure that the minister or chaplain has been called if the relatives wish

- Give an information or help leaflet to the relatives

- Notify the social worker if he or she is available

- Give useful telephone numbers and contact addresses (and your name) to the relatives

---

Other actions

Although they are stunned by events, it is often the small touches of care that relatives appreciate and remember, such as being given a lock of hair from their dead child by a thoughtful nurse.

Always ask if there is anyone else whom the relatives would like to be contacted—for example, a close friend or a minister. The hospital chaplains can be a source of great support to both relatives and busy staff.

If a mechanism of counselling and follow up exists locally consider borrowing their expertise in appropriate cases of trauma.

Sedation may be requested for relatives, usually by a third party but is generally inappropriate as it dulls reality and may delay acceptance. Grieving cannot be avoided so easily.

Leaflet explaining official procedures after death.

Follow up

Long term management and bereavement counselling is not within the scope of this article, but arrangements for follow up may need initiating on day one. If the nurse or doctor concerned in the emergency department feels able they can offer to see the relative again. Some departments have a social worker who can provide some practical help as well as coordinate follow up. Further information from necropsy may also be available. If death occurs it is helpful to have a routine checklist, which includes notifying the general practitioner.

An up to date leaflet explaining official procedures slipped into a relative's pocket is useful for later perusal (for example, leaflet D49, *What to do after Death*, which is published by the Department of Health). Participation by the coroner's officer, who may be a policeman, should be explained. Warning relatives of the possibility of them developing symptoms of post-traumatic stress disorder is appropriate in certain cases. (An explanatory leaflet that includes ways to get help would be useful in busy departments.) Such symptoms include depression, anxiety, and flash backs, with a wide range of severity. Also, it may be necessary in follow up to warn them of possible avoiding or unhelpful actions by neighbours. Details of any local organisations, such as CRUSE, from which help and practical advice can be obtained from trained counsellors, should also be given.

Difficulties for hospital staff in breaking bad news

- Lack of training and experience
- Fear of being blamed
- Not knowing how to cope with relatives' reactions
- Fear of expressing emotion
- Fear of not knowing the answers
- Fear of their own death or disability

Staff's reaction

Lastly, do not forget the carers. There are many different reactions, the commonest of which are sadness, anger, and guilt.[1] Staff may identify with particular people or situations. For example, a child being killed will be particularly upsetting, especially for staff with children of the same age. Part of the debriefing on major trauma must include an opportunity for members of staff to express their feelings. Hiding behind a defence of excessive concern with composure or tasks should be avoided.

Conclusion

National contact addresses

● **CRUSE** (for care of the bereaved) Cruse House, 126 Sheen Road, Richmond, Surrey TW9 1UR. Tel (071) 940 4818

● **Compassionate friends** (for bereaved parents) 6 Denmark Street, Bristol BS1 5DQ. Tel (0272) 292778

● **Foundation for the Study of Infant Deaths** 15 Belgrave Square, London SW1X 8PS. Tel (071) 235 1721

● **Samaritans** (for the despairing) 17 Uxbridge Road, Slough SL1 1SN. Tel (0753) 32713

1 Wright B. Sudden death: aspects which incapacitate the carer. *Nursing* 1988;**3**:12-5.
2 Buckman R. Breaking bad news: Why is it still so difficult? *BMJ* 1984;**288**:1597-9.

Further reading:
Kübler-Ross E. *On death and dying.* New York: MacMillan, 1969.
Wright B. *Sudden death.* Edinburgh: Churchill Livingstone, 1990.

Because of its suddeness and severity major trauma is especially difficult for relatives and staff to cope with. However bad the news is relatives need direct, honest information along with genuine understanding and support. Many doctors find this important part of their work difficult. Reasons have been suggested for this.[2] Awareness may help the situation and lead to a greater emphasis in training.

In short, the principles of dealing with the distressed relative can be remembered as follows:

● **Empathise.** Sit and listen to and reflect back relatives' reactions rather than make assumptions or categorise them

● **Enable** relatives to accept reality and to experience the pain

● **Encourage,** as in "you will be able to cope" (with help if needed)

● **Encounter** your own feelings and express them later, perhaps as part of a debriefing.

I thank Sister Susan Judge, Reverend Bob Irving, Dr Sheila Cassidy, and the staff of the accident and emergency department, Derriford Hospital, Plymouth, for ideas and advice; Jackie Eccleson for typing the manuscript; and the photographic department. I also thank the unfortunate relatives, whose reactions, comments, and questions have formed the basis of this article.

SCORING SYSTEMS FOR TRAUMA

D W Yates

Previous articles in this series have emphasised the importance of an aggressive, integrated, interdisciplinary approach to trauma care by an experienced team that has immediate access to operating theatres and intensive care facilities. Many of the recommendations can be expected to incur appreciable additional costs. Will this money be well spent? Which changes are most effective in improving patient care and are there any which produce unexpected delays or complications?

To answer these questions about a system which has to respond to patients with an almost infinite constellation of injuries is a major challenge in clinical measurement and audit. Clearly, statistical analysis must replace anecdote and dogma, but the complexity of the task should not be underestimated.

The effects of injury may be defined in terms of input—an anatomical component and the physiological response—and output—mortality and morbidity. These must be coded numerically before we can comment with confidence on treatment. Elderly people and young children survive trauma less well than others, so age must be taken into account. The mechanism of injury is also important: the effect of a blunt impact from a fall or a car crash is quite different from that of a stab or gunshot wound. Most recent work has been concerned with the measurement of injury severity and its relation to mortality. The assessment of morbidity has been largely neglected, yet there are two seriously impaired survivors for every person who dies owing to trauma.

Cost-benefit analysis of trauma care

Input
Anatomical injury
Physiological derangement

Treatment
Variations in the system of care
Variations in patient care

Output
Survival: alive or dead?
Disability: temporary or permanent?
   Neurological?
   Musculoskeletal?
   Visceral?

Input criteria

Examples of injuries scored by abbreviated injury scale

Injury	Score
Shoulder pain (no injury specified)	0
Wrist sprain	1 (Minor)
Closed undisplaced tibial fracture	2 (Moderate)
Head injury—unconscious on admission but for less than one hour thereafter, no neurological deficit	3 (Serious)
Major liver laceration, no loss of tissue	4 (Severe)
Incomplete transection of the thoracic aorta	5 (Critical)
Laceration of the brain stem	6 (Fatal)

Anatomical scoring system

The *abbreviated injury scale* (AIS) was first published in 1969. It scores from 1 (minor) to 6 (fatal) over 1200 injuries, which are listed in a booklet that is now in its fourth edition. (Copies of the booklet AIS90 may be obtained from the North Western Injury Research Centre—see footnote.) The intervals between the scores are not always consistent—for example, the difference between AIS3 and AIS4 is not necessarily the same as the difference between AIS1 and AIS2—but the higher the score the worse the injury.

Injury severity score

To obtain this:
(1) Use the AIS90 dictionary to score every injury
(2) Identify the highest abbreviated injury scale score in each of the following six areas: head and neck, abdomen and pelvic contents, bony pelvis and limbs, face, chest, and body surface
(3) Add together the squares of the three highest area scores

---

Patients with multiple injuries are scored by adding together the squares of the three highest abbreviated injury scale scores in predetermined regions of the body (see box). This is the *injury severity score* (ISS). The maximum score is 75 ($5^2+5^2+5^2$). By convention a patient with an AIS6 in one body region is given an injury severity score of 75. The injury severity score is non-linear: there is pronounced variation in the frequency of different scores—9 and 16 are common, 14 and 22 unusual, and 7 and 15 unattainable. The overall injury severity score of a group of patients should be identified by the median value and the range, not the mean value. Non-parametric statistics should be used for analyses.

Scoring systems for trauma

Case study

A man is injured in a fall at work. He complains of pain in his neck, jaw, and left wrist and has difficulty breathing. There are abrasions around the left shoulder, left side of the chest, and left knee. Examination of the cervical spine (with radiography) suggests no abnormality. There are fractures of the body of the mandible, left wrist, and left ribs (5 to 9), with a flail segment.

ISS=$2^2+2^2+4^2$=24

Injury	Abbreviated injury scale
Fracture of body of mandible	2
Fracture of lower end of radius (not further specified*)	2
Fracture of ribs 5-9 with flail segment	4
Abrasions (all sites)	1
Neck pain†	0

*If fracture of radius was known to be displaced or open the AIS would be 3. If not specified the lower score is used.

†Symptoms are not scored if there is no demonstrable anatomical injury.

Glasgow coma scale

	Score
Eyes open:	
Spontaneously	4
To speech	3
To pain	2
Never	1
Best motor response:	
Obeys commands	6
Localises pain	5
Flexion withdrawal	4
Decerebrate flexion	3
Decerebrate extension	2
No response	1
Best verbal response:	
Orientated	5
Confused	4
Inappropriate words	3
Incomprehensible sounds	2
Silent	1

Physiological scoring systems

The *Glasgow coma scale* (GCS) is the accepted international standard for measuring neurological state. The score may be represented as a single figure (for example, GCS=15) or as the response in each of the three sections (for example, eyes, motor response, and verbal response=465). Coma is defined as a Glasgow coma scale of <8.

Various modifications of the scale have been suggested for use in small children. Some doctors reduce the maximum score to that which is consistent with neurological maturation. A more useful clinical device, which ensures more accurate communication and simplifies epidemiological research is to retain the maximum score of 15 but to redefine the descriptions.

Modification of Glasgow coma scale for children

	Score
Best verbal response:	
Appropriate words or social smiles, fixes on and follows objects	5
Cries but is consolable	4
Persistently irritable	3
Restless, agitated	2
Silent	1
Eye and motor responses are scored as in scale for adults	

Revised trauma score

	Coded value	×weight	=score
Respiratory rate (breaths/min):			
10-29	4		
>29	3		
6-9	2	0.2908	_____
1-5	1		
0	0		
Systolic blood pressure (mm Hg):			
>89	4		
76-89	3		
50-75	2	0.7326	_____
1-49	1		
0	0		
Glasgow coma scale:			
13-15	4		
9-12	3		
6-8	2	0.9368	_____
4-5	1		
3	0		
			_____
Total=revised trauma score:			_____

The *revised trauma score* combines coded measurements of respiratory rate, systolic blood pressure, and Glasgow coma scale to provide a general assessment of physiological derangement. It was derived from statistical analysis of a large North American database to determine the most predictive independent outcome variables. Selection of variables was also influenced by their ease of measurement and clinical opinion. The coded value is multiplied by a weighting factor derived from regression analysis of the database. This correction reflects the relative value of the measurement in determining survival.

The injury severity score is often underestimated when the patient first arrives at hospital, and the revised trauma score changes as resuscitation progresses. For the purposes of the analyses described below the injury severity score should be calculated only from operative findings, appropriate investigations, or necropsy reports. The revised trauma score is, by convention, taken as the score recorded when the patient first arrives in the accident and emergency department.

TRISS methodology

TRISS methodology

Probability of survival of individual patient

$(Ps) = \dfrac{1}{1+e^{-b}}$

Where e = natural logarithm and $b = b_0 + b_1$ (RTS) $+ b_2$ (ISS) $+ b_3$ (A)

b_{0-3} = Weighted coefficients based on major trauma outcome study (United States) data. These differ for blunt and penetrating injuries

RTS = revised trauma score

ISS = injury severity score

A = age (score 0 if <54, score 1 if ≥55)

Injury severity match ("M" statistic)

Compares the range of injury severity in the sample population with that of the main database (range 0·00-1·00). Z statistic is invalid if M <0·88

Population outcome comparison ("Z" statistic)

Measures difference between actual and predicted number of deaths or survivors (range −1·96 to +1·96)

The degree of physiological derangement and the extent of the anatomical injury are measures of the threat to life. Mortality will also be affected by the age of the patient and by the method of wounding. A blunt assault produces different injury characteristics and physiological abnormalities than does a penetrating object.

The "TRISS methodology" combines the four elements—revised trauma score, injury severity score, age of the patient, and whether the injury is blunt or penetrating—to provide a measure of the probability of survival (Ps). (The acronym is tortuously developed from **TR**auma score and **I**njury **S**everity **S**core.) It is important to appreciate that Ps is merely a mathematical calculation; it is not an absolute measure of mortality but only of the probability of death. If a patient with a Ps of 80% dies the outcome is unexpected in that four out of five patients with such a Ps could be expected to survive. But the fifth would be expected to die—and this could be the patient under study. The use of charts to identify patients whose Ps lies on the "wrong side" of a line that represents 50% mortality is widespread but may lead to inappropriate conclusions being drawn about the care of individual patients if this point is not recognised. Such charts are helpful in identifying patients for discussion at audit meetings but should not be used as the sole measure of performance.

Hospital review

Example

St Elsewhere District General Hospital treated 311 patients in one year who fulfilled the entry requirements for the major trauma outcome study. The distribution of probability of survival estimates in these patients was compared with those in the United States database of 80 000 patients to provide the M statistic. In this case M = 0·94, signifying a patient population compatible with the main database. In all, 273 of the 311 patients survived. This compares with a prediction of 284 and gives a Z statistic of −4·81. A figure below −1·96 indicates an overall performance that is appreciably worse than expected.

Case study

A 65 year old pedestrian is knocked down, sustaining head, abdominal, and leg injuries. On arrival in the accident and emergency department he has a Glasgow coma score of 9, respiratory rate of 35 beats/min, and systolic blood pressure of 80 mm Hg. Computed tomography shows a small subdural haematoma with swelling of the left parietal lobe. There is a major laceration of the liver but no other intra-abdominal injury. Radiographs of the lower limbs show displaced fractures through both upper tibias.

Revised trauma score:

Glasgow coma score = 9; coded value 3 × weighting 0·9368 = 2·8104

Respiratory rate = 35; coded value 3 × weighting 0·2908 = 0·8724

Blood pressure = 80; coded value 3 × weighting 0·7326 = 2·1978

RTS = 5·8806

Injury severity score

	Abbreviated injury score
Subdural haematoma (small)	4
[Parietal lobe swelling]	[3]
Liver laceration (major)	4
Upper tibial fracture (displaced)	3

$ISS = 4^2 + 4^2 + 3^2 = 41$

Probability of survival

Coefficients from major trauma outcome study database for blunt injury:

$b_0 = -1·2470$

$b_1 = 0·9544$

$b_2 = -0·0768$

$b_3 = -1·9052$

$b = -1·2470 + (0·9544)(5·8806) + (-0·0768)(41) + (-1·9052)(1)$

$P_s = \dfrac{1}{1+e^{-(0·6886)}} = 0·3343$

Probability of survival = 33%

Major trauma outcome study

The major trauma outcome study

—Measures overall severity of injury

—Records management and outcome

—Provides a database for audit in individual patients

—Allows comparison of performance over time and between hospitals

---

First developed in North America, the method employed in the major trauma outcome study is now also used in the United Kingdom and Australia to audit the effectiveness of systems of trauma care and the management of individual patients. The TRISS methodology is applied in all patients with trauma who are admitted to hospital for more than three days, managed in an intensive care area, referred for specialist care, or die in hospital. Additional information is sought about pre-hospital care, the seniority of doctors attending the patient on arrival at hospital, the initial management, and the timing of consultations and operations.

Scoring systems for trauma

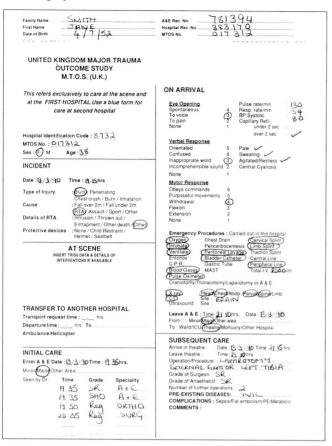

Form for recording patient's details at the scene and at the first hospital and outcome.

Output variables

> **Scoring systems should be developed to measure the quality of life after major trauma**

Measurement of the change in mortality that may occur in patients with a given combination of anatomical injury and physiological derangement is only one method of assessing the effects of modifications in the system of care. The quality of life of the survivors may vary considerably, but there is at present no adequate system of measuring this. The Glasgow outcome score is a recognised method for measuring the severity of permanent neurological impairment, but there is no universally accepted system for measuring disability resulting from injury to the musculoskeletal system. Most research has concentrated on the elderly and chronically infirm and has not addressed the issue of temporary disability that may be caused by injury to the locomotor system and incapacitate a young person for many months.

Future developments

Objectives of scoring systems

Short term objectives

- Better pre-hospital data
- Consistent hospital scoring
- Improved necropsy reports

Long term objectives

More sensitive scales to include:

- Biomechanical measurements
- More sensitive physiological assessment
- Biochemical analyses
- Assessment of temporary and permanent morbidity

There are wide variations in the provision of emergency medical services throughout the world, and the optimal system for the United Kingdom is still under debate. The major trauma outcome study provides an invaluable method for comparing the patterns of care in different parts of the country. This can be achieved only if data are carefully collected in a consistent format to allow collation and comparison of results. Deaths caused by trauma are too varied, too complicated, and too important to be discussed in isolation in individual hospitals, however sophisticated their software. The wide perspective of the major trauma outcome study is increasingly recognised as the only valid approach to trauma audit and is being taken up by regional and national bodies for this purpose. Identification of deficiencies is valuable, however, only if a mechanism exists to correct them. Local audit meetings and national comparisons must be used to stimulate appropriate changes in the systems of trauma care.

The development of the TRISS methodology has been a major advance in the measurement of injury severity. The detailed structure of the scales and the method of developing a single number to represent threat to life are, however, under constant review.

An alternative method of measuring anatomical injury has recently been described by using the root sum squares of the abbreviated injury scale scores of the head and trunk (anatomic profile). This has now been incorporated into a system for the characterisation of trauma (ASCOT), using different weightings for the revised trauma score and age.

These developments can be expected to lead to more accurate scoring systems, but for the present the TRISS methodology has a worldwide reputation for consistency and reasonable prediction of outcome. Immediate improvement in its usefulness could be made if, as is happening in some areas, ambulance crews measured the revised trauma score at the scene of the accident. This would allow a more scientific appraisal of the value of pre-hospital care. The accuracy of anatomical information could also be improved — particularly in necropsy reports: these are often inadequate for coding purposes and spinal cord injuries are rarely described in detail.

Measurement of outcome in terms of survival or death is, however, a crude yardstick. Further progress is required in measuring disability after non-cerebral injury. Most life threatening visceral injuries leave little disability. In contrast, musculoskeletal problems cause prolonged periods of disability and handicap. Some attempts have been made to measure permanent musculoskeletal sequelae, but the many more patients who sustain temporary incapacity are largely ignored in the statistics. Much more effort will be required to develop outcome measures based on disability; these are essential if the treatment of the multiply injured patient is to be based on sound scientific principles.

The latest edition of the *Abbreviated Injury Scale Booklet* (AIS90) and information about the major trauma outcome study (UK) is available from the North Western Injury Research Centre, University of Manchester, Hope Hospital, Salford M6 8HD.

Definitions of impairment, disability, and handicap

Impairment has an anatomical or physiological basis and is usually a consequence of musculoskeletal or cerebral injury (for example, an amputated finger, anosmia). It is easy to measure but variably related to the patient's activity

Disability is a functional consequence of an impairment so that the patient cannot perform activities of daily life. Its measurement is relevant to the patient's needs but it is influenced by the environment

Handicap refers to disability within the patient's social and professional environment. It reflects a change in lifestyle, but it is difficult to relate it to specific injury and is very difficult to measure

INDEX

Index

Index